CLASSIFICATION MANUAL
FOR
VOICE DISORDERS–I

CLASSIFICATION MANUAL
FOR
VOICE DISORDERS–I

Editors:
Katherine Verdolini, PhD, CCC-SLP
Clark A. Rosen, MD, FACS
Ryan C. Branski, PhD, CCC-SLP

Contributing authors (in alphabetical order):
Moya L. Andrews, PhD, CCC-SLP
Diane M. Bless, PhD, CCC-SLP
Daniel R. Boone, PhD, CCC-SLP
Janina K. Casper, PhD, CCC-SLP
Leslie E. Glaze, PhD, CCC-SLP
Michael Karnell, PhD, CCC-SLP
Christy L. Ludlow, PhD, CCC-SLP
Joseph C. Stemple, PhD, CCC-SLP

Other contributors (in alphabetical order):
Julie M. Barkmeier-Kraemer, PhD, CCC-SLP
Joseph Duffy, PhD, CCC-SLP
Rebecca J. Leonard, PhD, CCC-SLP
Rahul Shrivastav, PhD
Susan Thibeault, PhD, CCC-SLP

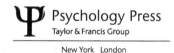

Psychology Press
Taylor & Francis Group

New York   London

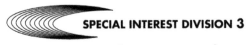

AMERICAN
SPEECH-LANGUAGE-
HEARING
ASSOCIATION

First pubished by

Lawrence Erlbaum Associates, Inc., Publishers
10 Industrial Avenue
Mahwah, New Jersey 07430

This edition published 2012 by Psychology Press

Psychology
Taylor & Francis Group
711 Third Avenue
New York, NY 10017

Psychology
Taylor & Francis Group
27 Church Road, Hove
East Sussex BN3 2FA

Cover design by Kathryn Houghtaling Lacey

Library of Congress Cataloging-in-Publication Data

Classification manual for voice disorders–I / editors, Katherine
Verdolini, Clark A. Rosen, Ryan C. Branski ; contributing
authors, Moya L. Andrews ... [et al.].
    p. cm.
Includes bibliographical references and index.
ISBN 0-8058-5631-5 (alk. paper)
1. Voice disorders—Classification—Handbooks, manuals, etc.
I. Verdolini, Katherine. II. Rosen, Clark A. III. Branski,
Ryan C. IV. Andrews, Moya L. V. American Speech-Lan-
guage- Hearing Association. Special Interest Division 3,
Voice and Voice Disorders.
RF510.C56   2005
616.85'5—dc22   2005047323
                                             CIP

DEDICATION

The *Classification Manual for Voice Disorders* is dedicated to four individuals whose contributions have been invaluable to the study and advancement of clinical voice science and management. Their records of excellence as scientists, clinicians, mentors, and colleagues have inspired and influenced the entire professional community of voice and voice disorders. The authors and editors of this document are delighted to dedicate this manual in their honor.

Daniel R. Boone, Speech–Language Pathologist

Dr. Boone has written, lectured, and taught for more than four decades in the area of voice disorders and voice therapy. His classic text, *The Voice and Voice Therapy*, is now in its seventh edition and remains the best selling and most widely read voice disorders textbook in the world. Dr. Boone combines his personable clinical approach with the best science and techniques available to produce favorable voice outcomes for his patients. His expertise is renowned as he has taught thousands of speech–language pathologists how to manage voice disorders. Ever the innovator, Dr. Boone's work with auditory feedback as a primary approach to voice therapy resulted in the development of Kay Elemetric's electronic instrument, the "Facilitator." Dr. Boone is also the author of a popular self-help text and audio compact disc entitled, *Is Your Voice Telling on You?* As a past President, Fellow, and Honoree of ASHA, and as a prolific author, lecturer, teacher, and advocate, the profession has benefited from Dr. Boone's visionary leadership and creative productivity. Recognizing Dr. Boone's many years of service and teaching to professionals in the area of voice and voice disorders, and his participation as an original author of this document, we dedicate this manual in his honor.

Janina Casper, Speech–Language Pathologist

Dr. Casper has made extensive and excellent contributions as a clinical researcher in voice disorders. Her colleagues, students, and patients commend her pragmatic approach to clinical problem solving. Indeed, she is the consummate clinical researcher; she cannot and will not separate these two significant components of her professional life. As a devoted and talented clinician, she has lectured nationally and internationally and is a co-presenter in the ASHA-sponsored video teaching tool, "Clinical Grand Rounds: Voice Disorders," a top-rated continuing education product for nearly a decade. Her research asks answerable questions, employs appropriate measures, and critically analyzes results to inform and improve the process of clinical voice management. Her collaborative publications helped define the utility of stroboscopy as a diagnostic tool and the importance of select instrumental measures in voice-disordered patients. Dr. Casper is a co-author of the popular graduate text, *Understanding Voice Problems: A Physiological Perspective for Diagnosis and Treatment.* She is a Fellow of ASHA and Professor Emeritus of Syracuse University. Throughout her career, Dr. Casper exhibited a fervent desire to bring order out of disorder, and her longstanding participation in the creation and editing of this classification document was a step toward that goal. We dedicate this manual in her honor.

Wilbur Gould, Otolaryngologist

Dr. Gould was a pre-eminent otolaryngologist and the founder of The Voice Foundation. Dr. Gould's sense of sharing and collaboration among and between all the professions dedicated to the care, understanding, treatment, and training of the voice was paramount. He was a constant role model for inclusion of those he believed could participate in making his patients better. In establishing The Voice Foundation, Dr. Gould brought together voice scientists, physicians, speech–language pathologists, acting coaches and singing teachers, and other professional voice users. Geographic boundaries posed no barrier and he actively sought out and recruited those throughout the world with an especial interest in voice. In his typical soft-spoken and self-effacing manner, he demonstrated how this networking of disciplines and worldviews could be of benefit to all. Dr. Gould had an abiding concern and interest in the variety of definitions, the unique jargon that professionals from these diverse yet overlapping disciplines used when perhaps speaking of the same thing. Recalling Dr. Gould's hope that an outgrowth of this collaborative approach would be a greater understanding of each other's jargon, a melding of terminology, and thereby a greater understanding of our combined expertise, we dedicate this manual in his memory.

G. Paul Moore

Dr. Moore is a historian, clinician, scientist, and mentor who has enriched the field of voice science and laid the cornerstone of our understanding of laryngeal physiology and its relationship to vocal pathology, vocal change, and gender. His classic high speed film of the larynx displayed a groundbreaking view of vocal fold vibration. In 1981, the board of directors of The Voice Foundation honored Dr. Moore by establishing the G. Paul Moore Lecture at the Annual Symposium: Care of the Professional Voice. This invited lectureship allows other accomplished scientists to share philosophical and historical perspectives on voice as Dr. Moore had always shared his knowledge. Dr. Moore is both a Fellow and an Honoree of ASHA. His work is also honored at the annual G. Paul Moore Symposium at the University of Florida, where Dr. Moore served as Department Chair in the Speech and Hearing Department from 1962–1973. He retired from academia in 1980, but never really stopped teaching and conducting research; in fact, he continues to influence the minds of students today. In the spirit of Dr. Moore's hope for state-of-the-art knowledge of voice science toward the goal of improving clinical care, we dedicate this manual in his honor.

Contents

Foreword

An original version of this manual was compiled in 1995 as an initiative of the American Speech–Language–Hearing Association Special Interest Division 3: Voice and Voice Disorders, under the direction of Dr. Christy Ludlow of the National Institutes of Health. Contributors were Drs. Moya Andrews, Diane Bless, Daniel Boone, Janina Casper, Leslie Glaze, Michael Karnell, Christy Ludlow, and Joseph Stemple. Dr. Rahul Shrivastav completed subsequent edits. The earlier versions of the manual established the overall structure of the document and laid the foundation for the present publication, which received extensive revision and expansion from a three-person collaborative editing team: Drs. Katherine Verdolini, Ryan Branski, and Clark Rosen (Otolaryngologist). In its final stages, this version received additional review and input from other contributors, including Drs. Julie Barkmeier-Kraemer, Joseph Duffy, Rebecca Leonard, and Susan Thibeault. Special Interest Division 3 acknowledges with gratitude the generous contributions of time and expertise provided by all of these participants. Their steadfast commitment to the completion of this project reflects their devotion to the advancement of interdisciplinary study and effective service delivery in voice and voice disorders.

Proceeds from the sale of this manual support the mission of Special Interest Division 3, which provides continuing education and networking opportunities to promote leadership and advocacy for issues in voice, addressed from professional, clinical, educational, and scientific perspectives. Affiliates of Special Interest Division 3 are members of ASHA who share a common interest in voice and voice disorders, including vocal development and lifespan changes, and the continuum of voice production from disordered through superior performance. This classification manual is the first reference of its kind in the field of voice disorders.

Overview and Purpose

The purpose of this manual is twofold. First, the manual is intended as a resource for information about conditions affecting voice. The intended audience is professionals working with voice disorders, including but not limited to speech–language pathologists, otolaryngologists, neurologists, and psychiatrists. Second, the manual is intended as a framework for classifying voice disorders, to facilitate communication among professionals in the assessment and management of patients with voice disorders.

The distinction between diagnosis and classification of a voice disorder is important. Diagnosis refers to the label that a qualified practitioner applies, indicating the presence of a given medical or other condition. Diagnoses are made by different practitioners depending on the condition: For example, otolaryngologists diagnose a vocal fold polyp, neurologists diagnose Parkinsonism, speech–language pathologists may diagnose Muscle Tension Dysphonia, and psychiatrists diagnose conversion disorder. On the other hand, *classification* of a voice disorder in this manual refers to the attribution of a voice problem to a specific class of disorders. Classification requires that consideration be given to the type of medical or other condition(s) that may play a role in a voice disorder, and the attributes of voice function that may be affected by the condition(s). Where individual practitioners may make diagnoses, classification may involve either an individual or a team of professionals.

Because voice function involves interaction among the laryngeal, respiratory, oral-pharyngeal, auditory, and somatosensory perception and cognitive systems, voice disorders can reflect a wide variety of different conditions, singly or in combination. It is recognized, therefore, that in many voice disorders, multiple factors play a role in voice dysfunction. Such factors may include present or previous medical condition(s), the patient's adjustment to these condition(s), and the patient's communication needs. Therefore, a medical diagnosis may only be one component in the classification of a patient's voice disorder when developing a plan for assessment and management of the problem by a multidisciplinary team.

CLARIFICATIONS

Inevitably, controversies exist about the essential nature of some of the conditions described in the manual. This situation reflects the dynamic and ongoing nature of advances in clinical and basic voice science, and also differences in clinical models used across clinicians. In its present form, the manual attempts to acknowledge controversies where they exist, and present alternative viewpoints that represent current knowledge and recognizable terms in the literature. One example of such controversy is whether nodules are properly diagnosed based on clinical inspection or findings from tissue biopsy. Another example is whether paresis can or should be diagnosed based on visual observations of decreased mobility. A third example involves voice disorders referred to as "functional."

Traditionally, functional voice disorder has been a diagnosis variably applied to patients with either presumed psychogenic laryngeal muscle adaptations or idiopathic etiology, in the absence of identifiable physical pathology. The terms *functional voice disorder* and *muscle tension dysphonia* have often been understood as diagnoses of exclusion. Clinical differentiation of specific psychogenic versus muscular indicators is rarely pursued and there are no empirical data to substantiate presumed muscular or functional adaptations that underlie dysphonia produced in the absence of organic etiology. This manual has employed the term Muscle Tension Dysphonia (Primary) (8010) to classify dysphonia that arises from apparent excessive use or misuse and hyper- or hypofunctional voice patterns in the absence of current organic vocal fold pathology, psychogenic, or neurologic etiology. Furthermore, we distinguish this primary dysphonia from a separate classification of Muscle Tension/Adaptive Dysphonia (Secondary) (8020), which describes the dysphonia that emerges secondarily in the presence of a current organic vocal fold pathology, psychogenic, or neurologic etiology. The term *adaptive* reflects the compensatory maladaptation to the primary etiology (e.g., change from normal or usual voice patterns in response to the primary condition) affecting voice production.

In summary, we have attempted to present state-of-the-art information relevant to voice disorders, some of which may challenge traditional concepts. Discussion is invited. The manual seeks to provide a common language for discussion, which can be considered and incorporated in future editions.

A final note relates to sources of information for the manual. Information was culled from personal discussions, extensive clinical experience, professional texts, reputable web-based information (e.g., emedicine.com), perceived consensus of specialists, and empirical data where available. Specific references as well as general resources are provided in the reference section of the manual.

SCOPE OF MANUAL

The manual lists most conditions that may negatively affect a patient's ability to produce voice, based on current understanding. It is anticipated that further entries will be added in later editions, and some of the current entries may be deleted. In all cases, a distinction is made between descriptions of the conditions themselves and their hypothesized effects on voice.

CLASSIFICATION SYSTEM CHARACTERISTICS

The system presented in this manual was loosely modeled after the *Diagnostic and Statistical Manual* (DSM) published by the American Psychiatric Association. Similar to the DSM system, the *Classification Manual of Voice Disorders-I (CMVD-I)* has been adapted to allow flexibility, and describe a large range of conditions affecting voice, while being simple for professionals to use. However, in contrast to the *DSM* series, the *CMVD-I* is not intended for diagnostic purposes. Rather, it is aimed at characterizing the condition(s) and dysfunction(s) involved in voice production. Moreover, the manual does not base disorder classifications on statistically derived categories. Also, major *axes* are not identified, delineating Clinical Disorders (Axis I) versus other aspects of functioning and health that may influence clinical course (Personality Disorders and Mental Retardation, Axis II, and General Medical Conditions, Axis III). Instead, the *CMVD-I* uses *dimensions*:

- *Dimension 1* pertains to the conditions involved in a current voice problem.
- *Dimension 2* codes the relative certainty of the current condition(s), in terms of both certainty of the medical or other conditions and certainty that the voice problem is attributable to the medical or other condition(s).

- *Dimension 3* codes the severity of the current condition in terms of both medical and vocal severity.
- *Dimension 4* codes the impact of a current voice problem on quality of life, from the patient's perspective.
- *Dimension 5* codes information about the current medical or other condition(s) and the voice problem, in the context of the overall clinical course (resolved, improving, stable, recurring, deteriorating).

DIMENSION 1. CATEGORIES OF CONDITIONS

CMVD-I Dimension 1 concerns the conditions that may contribute to a voice problem. Such conditions include structural pathologies, inflammation, trauma or injury, systemic disease, non-laryngeal aerodigestive disorders, psychiatric disorders, neurologic disorders, and conditions that are not otherwise specified. For each of these general classes of conditions, the manual provides information about specific issues, using the following organization:

Essential features: These are features that define the condition. For example, immobile vocal fold is an essential feature of unilateral vocal fold paralysis. In most cases, the condition is medical. Information is provided about the features expected in a particular medical or other condition.

Associated features: These are features that may accompany a condition, but are not essential features of it. For example, breathy voice may be associated with unilateral vocal fold paralysis. In most cases, associated features described in the manual are vocal, however, other associated features may also be described.

Vocal impairment: Information under this rubric describes general features of many voice problems associated with the condition. Information is provided about expected abnormalities based on acoustic, aerodynamic, and imaging observations, where such information is available.

Age at onset: Information is presented about the typical age at which signs or symptoms of the condition are first noted.

Course: Information is provided about the typical progression of the condition.

Complications: Information is provided about the most likely sequelae of the condition or its treatment.

Predisposing factors: In this section, information is provided about risk factors for the condition.

Frequency: Information is provided about how common the medical or other condition(s) are in the population at large. In almost all cases, information is lacking regarding frequency of voice problems due to the condition, but such information is included where available.

Sex ratio: This section indicates the distribution of the medical or other condition across males versus females.

Familial pattern: Here, information is provided about genetic or other familial factors in the condition.

Differential diagnosis: This section presents information about which other conditions must be ruled out, to increase confidence in the classification of what medical or other condition(s) may be involved. Information presented in this section is not intended to be exhaustive, but is indicative only. The physician involved with medical diagnosis will extend the considerations around differential diagnosis, depending on the circumstances.

Classification criteria: This section provides the essential criteria necessary for (a) identification of a condition in general, and (b) attribution of a voice problem to the condition(s). The establishment of a causal connection between a diagnostic condition and a voice problem is not always possible. Thus, when the patient is seen, the voice disorder has already developed and we can only see the outcome of the evolution of the disorder.

It may be helpful for practitioners to code all conditions possibly affecting voice using the numeric coding system provided (e.g. Vocal Fold Nodules = 1211). Examples are provided at the end of this introduction.

DIMENSION 2. LEVEL OF CLASSIFICATION CERTAINTY

After coding the presence of medical or other conditions that affect voice, the coder may use a numeric system to indicate the level of certainty for each condition (e.g. Systemic Lupus Erythematosus), and the attribution of a voice problem to that condition (e.g. episodic hoarseness). For both medical and vocal attributes, the following codings are suggested:

A. **Provisional Classification:** Insufficient information is available for classification. Future classification is unlikely without presentation of other signs or symptoms.

B. **Classification Deferred:** Insufficient information is available for classification. Future classification depends on clinical course or response to treatment.

C. **Provisional Classification Dependent Upon Diagnosis by the Appropriate Professional:** Sufficient information is available to make a working classification, however some degree of uncertainty persists (e.g. Systemic Lupus Erythematosus, provisional upon confirmation by blood work).

D. **Good Certainty of Classification Accuracy.**

E. **Certainty of Classification Accuracy.**

DIMENSION 3. CURRENT SEVERITY OF EACH CONDITION

After entering the code for classification certainty, the clinician may specify the current severity of each medical or other condition. Severity has two aspects, both of which are represented in parentheses. The first aspect reflects severity of the underlying disease or condition (e.g. Chronic Obstructive Pulmonary Disease). The second aspect of severity represents severity of the voice problem. The vocal severity rating should represent an integration of signs and symptoms as well as quality of life in relation to voice, as perceived by the clinician. Specific severity coding schemes are provided in the manual for conditions for which such schemes are widely used (e.g. Kashima Scale for Recurrent Respiratory Papilloma). Otherwise, the following general schemes can be used for medical or vocal severity:

> *Normal:* No signs, symptoms, or functional limitations.
> *Mild:* Limited signs, symptoms, or functional limitations.
> *Moderate:* Signs, symptoms, functional limitations between mild and severe.
> *Severe:* Significant signs, symptoms, or functional limitations.

DIMENSION 4. PATIENT-PERCEIVED IMPACT OF VOCAL FUNCTIONING ON QUALITY OF LIFE

The next dimension is a single score from a questionnaire that relates quality of life to voice. Two examples that have received particular examination in the literature are the *Voice Handicap Index* (VHI; Jacobson et al., 1997) and the *Voice-Related Quality-of-Life Measure* (*V-RQOL;*

Hogikyan & Sethuraman, 1999). Both of these tools are self-report questionnaires that reflect patients' perceptions of quality of life in relation to voice. The *VHI* has a total possible score of 120, whereas the *V-RQOL* has a possible score range of 10-50. Although higher raw scores imply worse function in the raw scores of both tools, the *V-RQOL* employs an algorithm that yields lower numerical values to reflect reduced quality of life related to voice. These scales and the scoring algorithms are provided in this manual.

DIMENSION 5. INFORMATION ABOUT CLINICAL COURSE

The final dimension provides information about clinical course. The coder may indicate information about the clinical course of the medical or other condition, and separately, about vocal function. Often, the clinical course may be similar across the condition and its associated vocal features. However, in other cases, the courses may differ.

- **R. Resolved:** This designation is used for medical or other conditions that have been present in the past, but are no longer operative. An example is vocal nodules, resolved after treatment.
- **I. Improving:** This designation indicates that the medical or vocal condition is generally improving.
- **S. Stable:** This designation indicates that the medical or vocal condition is generally stable, neither improving, deteriorating, nor cyclically recurring.
- **C. Cyclically Recurring:** This designation indicates a clinical course with intermittent recurrences.
- **D. Deteriorating:** This designation indicates a general clinical course that is in decline.

EXAMPLES OF USING THE CLASSIFICATION SYSTEM

Case 1 (pre-surgery):

A 45-year-old female teacher with a history of smoking presents with a mildly hoarse voice, and difficulty being understood in background noise. The otolaryngologic examination reveals a moderate-sized mid-fold lesion unilaterally, with stiff mucosa seen on stroboscopy. A cyst wall can be seen through the epithelium of the vocal fold. The patient is scheduled for laryngeal microsurgery for removal of the lesion. Coding for the current status of this patient is as follows:

Coding: 1213.C.D.(moderate, mild).VHI-37.S.S.
Explanation of code:

1213-Vocal Fold Cyst (Sub-epithelial)

C-Provisional diagnosis pending surgical confirmation

D-Good certainty that the mid-fold lesion affects the voice function; other factors may be smoking and environmental demands on voice function

Moderate-Describes the noted lesion

Mild-Describes severity of dysphonia

37-Score on the *VHI*

S-Stable medical condition

S-Stable voice condition prior to surgery

Case 1 (post surgery):

Following laryngeal microsurgery and voice therapy, repeated laryngeal examinations revealed smooth, straight vocal fold margins bilaterally, with good mucosal displacement characteristics. Also, repeated vocal function testing consistently revealed normal status. The patient had discontinued smoking, and used amplification in background noise. Coding for the patient's current condition is:

Coding: 1213.E.E.(normal, normal).VHI-8.S.S.
Explanation of coding:

1213-Although the original vocal fold cyst was successfully treated, that condition is nonetheless the reference for current evaluations

E-Diagnostic certainty is good

E-Certainty is also good that the normal voice status is related to good laryngeal status

Normal-Laryngeal appearance is normal

Normal-Vocal function is normal

8-Score on the *VHI*

S-The laryngeal condition is stable

S-The vocal condition is stable

Case 2 (post Botox® treatment):

> An otherwise healthy 37-year-old male presented with intermittent voice breaks and strain. Clinical testing ruled out essential tremor, sustained hyperfunction, and abductory spasms. A neurologist also confidently ruled out other neurologic conditions. The patient responded to botulinum toxin A injection to the thyroarytenoid/lateral cricoarytenoid complex with good resolution of symptoms for 3 to 4 months following injection, after which time he experienced gradual symptom recurrence. The current evaluation showed both a strained, tight voice quality and moderate voice spasms during all-voiced running speech. Current coding for this patient is:

> *Coding:* 7210.E.E.(moderate, moderate).*V-RQOL*-36.S.S.

> **7210-**Adductor spasmodic dysphonia

> **E-**No history or other neurologic findings suggest no contribution of other conditions, thus certainty of classification accuracy is excellent for the medical diagnosis

> **E-**No findings suggest no contribution of other conditions to the voice problem, thus there is excellent certainty in attributing the problem to adductor spasmodic dysphonia

> **Moderate-**Describes vocal fold movement abnormalities during speech

> **Moderate-**Describes vocal signs of breaks during vowels and hoarseness

> **36-**Raw score on *V-RQOL*

> **S-**Vocal fold movement abnormalities are recurring

> **S-**Vocal signs are recurring

Case 3 (evaluation):

> A 27-year-old female presented with substantial verbal hostility and frustration over her voice condition. She related a 5-year history of intermittent raspy voice corresponding to extreme fatigue accompanied by mild fever. Fever usually resolved after about 24 to 36 hours, however, voice problems and extreme fatigue persisted for up to 3 weeks. Fatigue never completely resolved. Numerous prior examinations by multiple practitioners had not led to any clear diagnosis or improvement in the condition. The patient denied odynophonia during symptomatic period; she also denied classic reflux symptoms

(e.g., heartburn, belching, bitter taste in mouth). The patient declared she was in good health otherwise, and had not sought medical attention for other conditions. However, she mentioned a recent finding of positive antinuclear antibody tests, which was confirmed by the medical records. A rheumatologist was monitoring her condition, and had scheduled follow-up tests in 3 months. Initial laryngeal examination, conducted while the patient was symptomatic, revealed moderate diffuse posterior laryngeal edema. Voice tests during a symptomatic phase revealed extreme hoarseness and diplophonia, which did not respond to stimulability testing. Voice during non-symptomatic phases was entirely normal. An appropriate coding for this patient is:

Coding: 2300.B.B.(moderate, moderate).59.C.C.
           4240.C.B.(mild, moderate).59.C.C.

Explanation of coding:

2300-Laryngopharyngeal Reflux

B-Classification deferred pending observation regarding clinical course and response to treatment

B-Poor certainty that the patient's voice complaints are due to Laryngopharyngeal Reflux. The patient's response to anti-reflux medications may alter the certainty

Moderate-Describes laryngeal signs of possible Reflux

Moderate-Describes overall voice function

59-Score on VHI

C-Describes cyclical recurrence of laryngeal signs

C-Describes cyclical recurrence of vocal signs

4240-Systemic Lupus Erythematosus

C-Provisional diagnosis; awaiting further testing

B-Some certainty that this condition may be contributing to the voice complaints

Mild-Describes severity of disease

Moderate-Describes severity of vocal signs

59-Score on VHI

C-Describes cyclical recurrence of the disease process

C-Describes cyclical recurrence of vocal signs

Follow-up note:

The patient's hostile and argumentative attitude, together with non-specific complaints not readily corresponding to an obvious laryngeal pathology, could be misleading. Classification of a voice problem as psychological requires positive evidence of a specific mental diagnosis, as well as suggested causal links between the diagnosis and voice. Because such evidence was lacking in this patient's case, it would not meet the criteria for a "psychological" condition.

Case 4 (post treatment):

An 82-year-old male suffered an infarct of the left middle cerebral artery (MCA) 6 months prior to presentation in the voice clinic. Primary functional sequelae of that stroke included dysarthria, aphasia, and right hemiplegia. The patient's presentation in the voice clinic indicated a 2-month history of hoarseness unassociated with other upper respiratory involvement. He declared a history of smoking 50 packs a year together with consumption of 5 to 10 shots of whiskey daily. Initial otolaryngological examination revealed a suspicious left vocal fold lesion involving the anterior commissure. Microlaryngoscopy and biopsy subsequently confirmed the presence of abnormal squamous cell invasion extending through the lamina propria, unilaterally. He was found to be negative for both cervical lymph node and distant metastasis. The lesion was removed during subsequent microlaryngoscopy, the margins were clear, and both post-operative larynx and voice appeared healthy and normal at a 3-week follow-up. Speech remained mildly dysarthric, and mild Broca's aphasia persisted. The appropriate coding for this patient is:

Coding: 1110.E.D.(T1.N0.M0, normal).32.R.R.
　　　　Speech condition is noted separately as: S/p MCA infarct; dysarthria, aphasia.
Explanation of coding:

1110-Malignant lesion of the left vocal fold

E-No findings have been seen suggesting the contribution of other conditions, thus certainty of classification accuracy is excellent for the medical diagnosis

D-There is good certainty in attributing the problem to the vocal fold lesion. Dysarthria may also be contributing to voice function for speech communication

T1.N0.M0-Established severity scale for malignant lesions

Normal-Voice was normal, although dysarthria was evident in other aspects of speech production

32-Raw Score on V-RQOL; this score might be confounded by the patient's difficulty distinguishing the functional impact of speech dysarthria on quality-of-life ratings for voice

R-Laryngeal disease resolved

R-Voice signs resolved; speech dysarthria is noted separately

Note: The patient's other medical condition, status-post MCA infarct with current mild dysarthria and mild Broca's aphasia, does not appear contributory to the laryngeal or vocal situation. Thus, although these conditions are present, they are not coded using the voice classification scheme but are noted descriptively.

Case 5 (post therapy):

A 63-year-old female has a long-standing diagnosis of Parkinson disease. The condition continues to progress, to the point where the woman is now considered to have Hoehn and Yahr Stage 3 disease. Otolaryngological examination reveals a mild spindle-shaped gap between the vocal folds that was eliminated during effortful voice production. The patient recently underwent a full course of Lee Silverman Voice Treatment (Ramig, Countryman, O'Brien, Hoehn, & Thompson, 1996). The patient's voice output improved from an average of 65 dB at 30 cm prior to treatment, to an average of 75 dB at 30 cm after treatment, during most spontaneous speech. The speech–language pathologist considers that the patient has a mild residual voice problem, improved from moderate or severe prior to treatment. The appropriate coding is:

Coding: 7420.E.E.(moderate, mild).33.D.I.
Explanation of coding:

7420-Parkinson disease as diagnosed by a neurologist

E-No findings have been seen suggesting the contribution of other conditions, thus certainty of classification accuracy is excellent for the medical diagnosis

E-No findings suggest a contribution of other conditions to the voice problem, thus there is excellent certainty in attributing the problem to Parkinson disease

Moderate-Describes the severity of the disease

Mild-Describes the severity of the voice; dysarthria is noted separately

33-Score on VHI

D-Describes medical condition as deteriorating

I-Describes general improvement of vocal function; dysarthria is noted separately

Name: _____ Date: _____

VOICE HANDICAP INDEX

Jacobson, Johnson, Grywalski, Silbergleit, Jacobson, Benninger, & Newman, 1997*

Instructions: These are statements that many people have used to describe their voices and the effects of their voices on their lives. Circle the response that indicates how frequently you have the same experience.

0 = Never 1 = Almost Never 2 = Sometimes 3 = Almost Always 4 = Always

Part I (F = Functional)

1) My voice makes it difficult for people to hear me.	0 1 2 3 4
2) People have difficulty understanding me in a noisy room.	0 1 2 3 4
3) My family has difficulty hearing me when I call them throughout the house.	0 1 2 3 4
4) I use the phone less often than I would like.	0 1 2 3 4
5) I tend to avoid groups of people because of my voice.	0 1 2 3 4
6) I speak with friends, neighbors, or relatives less often because of my voice.	0 1 2 3 4
7) People ask me to repeat myself when speaking face-to-face.	0 1 2 3 4
8) My voice difficulties restrict personal and social life.	0 1 2 3 4
9) I feel left out of conversations because of my voice.	0 1 2 3 4
10) My voice problem causes me to lose income.	0 1 2 3 4

Part II (P = Physical)

1) I run out of air when I talk.	0 1 2 3 4
2) The sound of my voice varies throughout the day.	0 1 2 3 4
3) People ask, "What's wrong with your voice?"	0 1 2 3 4
4) My voice sounds creaky and dry.	0 1 2 3 4

5) I feel as though I have to strain to produce voice.   0 1 2 3 4

6) The clarity of my voice is unpredictable.   0 1 2 3 4

7) I try to change my voice to sound different.   0 1 2 3 4

8) I use a great deal of effort to speak.   0 1 2 3 4

9) My voice is worse in the evening.   0 1 2 3 4

10) My voice "gives out" on me in the middle of speaking.   0 1 2 3 4

Part III (E = Emotional)

1) I am tense when talking with others because of my voice.   0 1 2 3 4

2) People seem irritated with my voice.   0 1 2 3 4

3) I find other people don't understand my voice problem.   0 1 2 3 4

4) My voice problem upsets me.   0 1 2 3 4

5) I am less outgoing because of my voice problem.   0 1 2 3 4

6) My voice makes me feel handicapped.   0 1 2 3 4

7) I feel annoyed when people ask me to repeat.   0 1 2 3 4

8) I feel embarrassed when people ask me to repeat.   0 1 2 3 4

9) My voice makes me feel incompetent.   0 1 2 3 4

10) I am ashamed of my voice problem.   0 1 2 3 4

*Jacobson B, Johnson A, Grywalski C, Silbergleit A, Jacobson G, Benninger M, & Newman, C (1997). The voice handicap index (VHI): development and validation. *American Journal of Speech Language Pathology, 6,* 66–70.

Name: _____ Date: _____

VOICE-RELATED QUALITY OF LIFE MEASURE (V-RQOL)

Hogikyan & Sethuraman, 1999*

We are trying to learn more about how a voice problem can interfere with your day-to-day activities. On this paper, you will find a list of possible voice-related problems. Please answer all questions based upon what your voice has been like over the past **two weeks**. There are no "right" or "wrong" answers. Considering both how severe the problem is when you get it, and how frequently it happens, please rate each item below on how "bad" it is (that is, the **amount** of each problem that you have). Use the following scale for rating the **amount** of the problem:

1 = None, not a problem
2 = A small amount
3 = A moderate (medium) amount
4 = A lot
5 = Problem is as "bad as it can be"

Because of my voice, how much of a problem is this?

1. I have trouble speaking loudly or being heard in noisy   1 2 3 4 5
   situations.

2. I run out of air and need to take frequent breaths when talking. 1 2 3 4 5

3. I sometimes do not know what will come out when I   1 2 3 4 5
   being speaking.

4. I am sometimes anxious or frustrated (because of my voice). 1 2 3 4 5

5. I sometimes get depressed (because of my voice).   1 2 3 4 5

6. I have trouble using the telephone (because of my voice).   1 2 3 4 5

7. I have trouble doing my job or practicing my profession   1 2 3 4 5
   (because of my voice).

8. I avoid going out socially (because of my voice).   1 2 3 4 5

9. I have to repeat myself to be understood.   1 2 3 4 5

10. I have become less outgoing (because of my voice).   1 2 3 4 5

1. V-RQOL General Scoring Algorithm:

$$100 - \frac{(\text{Raw Score - \# items in domain or total})}{(\text{Highest possible Raw Score} - \text{\# items})} \times 100$$

2. Social–Emotional Domain (Items 4, 5, 8, 10):

$$100 - \frac{(\text{Raw Score} - 4)}{16} \times 100$$

3. Physical Function Domain (Items 1, 2, 3, 6, 7, 9):

$$100 - \frac{(\text{Raw Score} - 6)}{24} \times 100$$

4. Total Score (Items 1–10):

$$100 - \frac{(\text{Raw Score} - 10)}{40} \times 100$$

Example for Total Score

If Raw Score is 30 (such as if a "medium problem" exists with all items), then:

$$100 - \frac{(20)}{40} \times 100 = 100 - (0.5 \times 100) = 100 - 50 = 50 \text{ Standard Score}$$

*Hogikyan ND, Sethuraman G. Validation of an instrument to measure Voice-Related Quality of Life (V-RQOL). *J Voice.* 1999;13:557–569. Reprinted from *Journal of Voice* with permission from The Voice Foundation.

1000. STRUCTURAL PATHOLOGIES OF THE LARYNX

1100. Malignant Laryngeal Lesions

1110. Malignant Vocal Fold Lesions

1120. Dysplasia/carcinoma in situ

1130. Laryngeal Malignancy (Non-Vocal Fold Origin)

1200. Epithelial and Lamina Propria Abnormalities of the Vocal Fold

1210. Focal Benign Lesions of the Lamina Propria

1211. Vocal Fold Nodules

1212. Fibrous Mass–Sub-Epithelial

1213. Fibrous Mass–Ligament

1214. Vocal Fold Polyp(s)

1215. Vocal Fold Cyst–Sub-Epithelial

1216. Vocal Fold Cyst–Ligament

1217. Reactive Vocal Fold Lesion

1220. Reinke's Edema

1230. Vocal Fold Scar

1231. Vocal Fold Scar Proper

1232. Vocal Fold Sulcus

1240. Vocal Fold Granuloma

1241. Non-Intubation Related Vocal Fold Granuloma

1242. Intubation Related Vocal Fold Granuloma/Contact Ulcer

1250. Keratosis (Sometimes Described as Leukoplakia or Erythroplasia)

1260. Recurrent Respiratory Papillomatosis (RRP)

1270. Subglottic Stenosis

1280. Acquired Glottic/Laryngeal Stenosis (Anterior Glottic Web)

1300. Vascular Abnormalities of the Vocal Fold

1310. Vocal Fold Hemorrhage

1320. Varix and Ectasia of the Vocal Fold

1400. Congenital and Maturational Changes Affecting Voice

1410. Congenital Webs (Synechia)

1420. Cri du Chat Syndrome

1430. Laryngomalacia

1440. Puberphonia

1450. Presbyphonia

2000. INFLAMMATORY CONDITIONS OF THE LARYNX

2100. Cricoarytenoid and Cricothyroid Arthritis

2200. Acute Laryngitis

2300. Laryngopharyngeal Reflux

2400. Chemical Sensitivity/Irritable Larynx Syndrome

3000. TRAUMA OR INJURY OF THE LARYNX

3100. Internal Laryngeal Trauma

3110. Laryngeal Mucosa Trauma (Chemical and Thermal)

3120. Intubation/Extubation Injuries of the Laryngeal Mucosa

3130. Arytenoid Dislocation

3200. External Laryngeal Trauma

4000. SYSTEMIC CONDITIONS AFFECTING VOICE

4100. Endocrine

4110. Hypothyroidism

4120. Hyperthyroidism

4130. Sexual Hormone Imbalances

4140. Growth Hormone Abnormalities (Hyperpituitarism)

4200. Immunologic

4210. Allergic Diseases of the Upper Respiratory Tract

4220. HIV and AIDS

4230. Chronic Fatigue Syndrome

4240. Systemic Lupus Erythematosus

4250. Sjogren's Syndrome

4260. Scleroderma

4270. Wegener's Disease

4300. Musculo-Skeletal Conditions Affecting Voice

  4310. Overuse Injury and Repetitive Strain Injury

  4320. Fibromyalgia

  4330. Ehler Danlos Syndrome

4400. Dehydration

5000. NON-LARYNGEAL AEROGESTIVE DISORDERS AFFECTING VOICE

  5100. Respiratory Diseases Affecting Voice

    5110. Asthma

    5120. Chronic Obstructive Pulmonary Disease

  5200. Digastric

    5210. Gastroesophageal Reflux Disease

  5300. Infectious Diseases of the Aerodigestive Tract

    5305. Laryngotracheobronchitis (Croup)

    5310. Pertussis (Whooping cough)

    5315. Diphtheria

    5320. Pneumonia

    5325. Infectious Sinusitis

    5330. Tuberculosis

    5335. Upper Respiratory Infection (URI)

    5340. Acute Epiglottitis

5345. Syphilis

5350. Sarcoidosis

5355. Scleroma of the Larynx (Klebsiella Rhinoscleromatis)

5360. Leprosy (Affecting the Larynx)

5365. Actinomycosis

5400. Mycotic (Fungal) Infections

5410. Blastomycosis

5420. Histoplasmosis

5430. Candidiasis

5440. Coccidioidomycosis (Valley Fever, Desert Fever,
San Joaquin Fever)

6000. PSYCHIATRIC AND PSYCHOLOGICAL DISORDERS
AFFECTING VOICE

6010. Somatoform Disorders

6011. Somatization Disorder

6012. Conversion Disorder

6013. Pain Disorder

6014. Hypochondriasis

6020. Factitious Disorder

6030. Selective Mutism

6040. Anxiety

6041. Posttraumatic Stress Disorder

6042. Generalized Anxiety Disorder

6050. Mood Disorders

6051. Major Depressive Disorder (Recurrent)

6052. Bipolar I Disorder

6060. Gender Identity Disorder

6070. Psychogenic Polydipsia

6080. Psychogenic Tremor-Like Voice Fluctuations

7000. NEUROLOGIC DISORDERS AFFECTING VOICE

7100. Peripheral Nervous System Pathology

7110. Superior Laryngeal Nerve (SLN) Pathology

7120. Unilateral Recurrent Laryngeal Nerve (RLN) Paralysis

7130. Unilateral or Bilateral Recurrent Laryngeal Nerve (RLN) Paresis

7140. Bilateral Recurrent Laryngeal Nerve (RLN) Paralysis–Peripheral

7150. Myasthenia Gravis

7160. Peripheral Neuropathy (Neuropathy, Charcot Marie Tooth or hereditary motor and sensory neuropathy)

7170. Enhanced Physiologic Tremor Affecting Voice

7200. Movement Disorders Affecting the Larynx

7210. Adductor Spasmodic Dysphonia

7220. **Abductor Spasmodic Dysphonia**

7230. **Mixed Abductor/Adductor Spasmodic Dysphonia**

7240. **Dystonic Tremor Affecting Voice**

7250. **Essential Tremor Affecting Voice**

7260. **Meige's Syndrome (Orofacial dystonia)**

7270. **Tardive Stereotypies (Tardive Dyskinesia)**

7280. **Tourette's Syndrome**

7300. **CENTRAL NERVOUS SYSTEM DISTURBANCE**

7305. **Amyotrophic Lateral Sclerosis (ALS; Lou Gehrig's Disease)**

7310. **Wallenberg Syndrome (Lateral Medullary Syndrome/ Infarct)**

7315. **Parkinson Disease**

7320. **Multiple Systems Atrophy (Shy-Drager Syndrome, Striatonigral Degeneration, Sporadic Olivoponto-cerebellar Atrophy)**

7325. **Progressive Supranuclear Palsy (Includes Pseudobulbar Palsy and Steele-Richardson-Olszewski Syndrome)**

7330. **Multiple Sclerosis**

7335. **Cerebellar Disorders**

7340. **Huntington's Chorea**

7345. **Bilateral Recurrent Laryngeal Nerve Paralysis–Central**

7350. **Myoclonus**

8000. OTHER DISORDERS AFFECTING VOICE

8010. Muscle Tension Dysphonia (Primary)

8020. Muscle Tension/Adaptive Dysphonia (Secondary)

8030. Ventricular Dysphonia

8040. Paradoxical Vocal Fold Movement Disorder (Vocal Cord Dysfunction)

9000. VOICE DISORDERS: UNDIAGNOSED OR NOT OTHERWISE SPECIFIED (NOS)

1000. STRUCTURAL PATHOLOGIES OF THE LARYNX

1100. Malignant Laryngeal Lesions

1110. Malignant Vocal Fold Lesions

Essential features. The majority of malignancies of the vocal folds involve abnormalities of the squamous cell epithelial lining. Squamous cell cancer of the vocal fold is defined by invasive growth from the epithelium to deeper structures of the vocal folds including the lamina propria and the vocalis muscle. Such cancers typically begin unilaterally but can extend to the opposite vocal fold. Rarely do laryngeal cancers derive from other tissues. Examples of such rare cases include connective tissue sarcomas, adenocarcinomas, lymphomas, etc.

Associated features. Hoarseness is a presenting symptom, and may be due to mass and stiffness changes in the vocal folds, irregular margins, and possible fixation. The degree of voice impairment is related to the size of the lesion, its location, and the degree of tissue invasion. Voice quality, therefore, may range from slight dysphonia to severe dysphonia or aphonia. Other associated features may include swallowing difficulty, weight loss, chronic cough, fetid breath, hemoptysis (coughing blood), otalgia, inhalation stridor and dyspnea.

Vocal impairment. Voice lab findings vary based on the characteristics of the pathology.

Aerodynamic characteristics. Minimum and average phonatory airflows may be increased if lesions limit vocal fold closure, or decrease if lesions obstruct airway.

Acoustic characteristics. Perturbation may be increased, and signal-to-noise ratio may be decreased, depending on lesion characteristics.

Age at onset. Usually between 60 to 70 years, but has been known to occur in the very young and the very old.

Course. Tumors are thought to begin as small lesions of the epithelium (carcinoma in situ), and when left untreated, will invade the deeper structures of the vocal fold. The lesions begin as unilateral, but may spread to involve both folds. Without medical or surgical treatment, malignant vocal fold lesions are life threatening.

Complications. Hoarseness is the only complication of early stage malignant vocal fold lesions. As the lesion progresses, so does the degree of hoarseness and the likelihood of dysphagia and compromised airway. Cancers that are left untreated, or are advanced, typically metastasize to regional cervical lymph nodes and possibly distant organs (lung, liver, spleen, skin, brain). The ultimate consequence is death.

Predisposing factors. Smoking and alcohol abuse are the most often cited factors associated with the development of all laryngeal carcinomas. Some data indicate a role of previous radiotherapy to the neck, dietary deficiencies, and exposure to environmental carcinogenic agents, e.g. asbestos, in some cases. Recently, some literature associated extraesophageal reflux disease with laryngeal carcinoma, but there is continued controversy over the relation between reflux and laryngeal cancer. Links have also been made between laryngeal cancer and human papilloma virus.

Frequency. Laryngeal cancers are reported to be between 2% of all cancers in women and 5% of all malignancies in men.

Sex ratio. The ratio of men to women who develop malignant laryngeal lesions is 4–5: 1, with the ratio narrowing steadily over the past 20 years.

Familial pattern. Unknown.

Differential diagnosis. Benign lesions of the vocal fold (papilloma, granuloma), infection (tuberculosis, fungal, etc.), amyloidosis, keratosis, Wegener's Granulomatosis, rheumatoid arthritis, and lymphoma.

Classification criteria.

(a) Required for medical diagnosis: Confirmation of malignancy through biopsy and histological analysis (abnormal cell invasion of lamina propria and/or muscle).

(b) Required to attribute a voice problem to the medical diagnosis: Voice disorder not wholly explained by other causes.

Severity criteria
(AJCC Cancer Staging Manual, 6th edition, 2002).

(a) Medical:

Tis: Carcinoma in situ. Cancer cells do not extend beyond epithelium.

T1: Tumor limited to the vocal fold(s), which may involve the anterior or posterior commissures, with normal vocal fold mobility.

    T1a: Tumor limited to one vocal fold.

    T1b: Tumor involves both vocal folds.

T2: Tumor extends to the supraglottis and/or subglottis, and/or there is impaired vocal fold mobility.

T3: Tumor limited to the larynx with vocal fold fixation or present in the base of tongue.

T4: Tumor invades through the thyroid cartilage and/or extends to other tissues beyond the larynx (e.g., pharynx, trachea, thyroid, esophagus, base of tongue).

NX: Regional lymph nodes cannot be assessed.

N0: No regional lymph node metastasis.

N1: Metastasis in a single ipsilateral lymph node 3 cm or less in greatest dimension.

N2: Metastasis in a single ipsilateral lymph node, more than 3 cm but less than 6 cm in greatest dimension; or in multiple ipsilateral lymph nodes, none more than 6 cm in greatest dimension; or in bilateral or contralateral lymph nodes, none more than 6 cm in greatest dimension.

N2a: Metastasis in a single ipsilateral lymph node, more than 3 cm but less than 6 cm in greatest dimension.

N2b: Metastasis in multiple ipsilateral lymph nodes, none more than 6 cm in greatest dimension.

N2c: Metastasis in bilateral or contralateral lymph nodes, none more than 6 cm in greatest dimension.

N3: Metastasis in a lymph node more than 6 cm in greatest dimension.

MX: Distant metastases cannot be assessed.

M0: Distant metastases not present.

M1: Distant metastases present.

Used with permission of the American Joint Committee on Cancer (AJCC), Chicago, Illinois. The original source for this material is the AJCC Cancer Staging Manual, 6th edition (2002), published by Springer-Verlag, New York, www.springeronline.com.

(b) Vocal: See Introduction.

1120. Dysplasia/carcinoma in situ

Essential features. Dysplasia (abnormal cell development) is a process of qualitative changes in the direction of malignancy in the appearance of epithelial cells. Carcinoma in situ involves malignant degeneration of epithelial cells that have not invaded outside of their native location. Malignant cells replace all layers of the epithelium. The differentiation between different grades of dysplasia and carcinoma in situ can only be made using light microscopy.

Associated features. Voice disruption is often present due to increased stiffness of the vocal fold cover.

Vocal impairment. Voice may be normal or near normal, or may be more severely affected. "Raspiness" is a typical characteristic when dysphonia is present.

Aerodynamic characteristics. Minimum and average phonatory airflows may be increased if lesions limit vocal fold closure or decreased if lesions obstruct the airway.

Acoustic characteristics. Perturbation may be increased, and signal-to-noise ratio may be decreased, depending on lesion characteristics.

Age at onset. Adulthood, most frequently occurring between the ages of 40 and 60 years.

Course. The course can be variable, in that lesions may be stable over time, without change, or they can progress in the dimensions of size, regional spread, or become carcinomas. Behavioral therapy may be helpful following or during medical or surgical treatment for optimization of voice and swallowing functions.

Complications. The primary complication is the progression to invasive carcinoma.

Predisposing factors. These may include chronic irritations from chemicals and tobacco smoke, alcohol, and laryngopharyngeal reflux.

Frequency. The yearly occurrence of laryngeal carcinoma in situ is 0.4/100,000 in the general population.

Sex ratio. Frequency appears higher in males.

Familial pattern. Unknown.

Differential diagnosis. Keratosis (keratin in epithelium), invasive carcinoma, and other vocal fold lesions. Also infectious processes, such as candida, must be ruled out.

Classification criteria.

(a) Required for medical diagnosis:

I. Dysplasia

Atypical cytological features in the laryngeal squamous epithelium without histopathologic evidence of malignancy (see Malignant Lesions of the Larynx).

II. Carcinoma in situ

Presence of cells that are non-stratified and undifferentiated, occupying a region ranging from more than two thirds to the full thickness of the epithelium. An associated feature is usually obvious nuclear pleomorphism (change in nuclear shape or size from cell to cell) including oddly shaped large nuclei.

(b) Required to attribute a voice problem to the medical diagnosis:
Voice changes that vary depending on the specific nature of the physical problem, attributable to the identified lesions, not wholly explained by other causes.

Severity criteria.

(a) Medical:

Mild/minimal dysplasia: Minimal but demonstrable changes in cellular structures. Stratification of the squamous epithelium is preserved, and cytoplasmic differentiation of the superficial layers is seen, with easily visible intracellular bridges and keratinization.

Moderate dysplasia: Undifferentiated cells extend to two thirds of the thickness of the epithelium. Differentiation and stratification are still seen in the superficial third of the epithelium.

Severe dysplasia or carcinoma in situ: Non-stratified, undifferentiated cells occupy regions ranging from over two thirds of the epithelium up to its full thickness. Three stages of carcinoma in situ have been previously distinguished.

(b) Vocal: See Introduction

1130. Laryngeal Malignancy (Non-Vocal Fold Origin)

Essential features. Invasion of epithelial cells into deeper tissue layers, anywhere within the larynx but not involving the true vocal folds. The most common sites are the ventricular folds, epiglottis, and pyriform sinuses. Lesions are usually identified later in the course of development as their increased size begins to interfere with voice, swallowing, or breathing.

Associated features. Hoarseness may result when the lesion interferes with airflow or when the mass interferes with the movement of one or both vocal folds. The malignancy may extend deep into the larynx, limiting vocal fold mobility. Swallowing difficulties, breathing difficulties, weight loss, fetid breath, pain in the throat, and ear pain may occur.

Vocal impairment. The degree of vocal impairment is related to the size of the lesion and its effects on respiration and movement of the vocal folds. Voice quality, therefore, may range from unimpaired to severely impaired depending on the size and location of the lesion. Voice lab test results vary with the same factors.

Aerodynamic characteristics. Minimum and average phonatory airflows may be increased if lesions limit vocal fold closure or decreased if lesion limits airway size.

Acoustic characteristics. Perturbation may be increased, and signal-to-noise ratio may be decreased, depending on lesion characteristics.

Age at onset. Typically a disease of adulthood.

Course. The lesion begins as a small abnormality of the epithelium and if left untreated will invade the deeper structures of the larynx. Without medical or surgical treatment, malignant laryngeal lesions are life threatening. Behavioral therapy is often required following medical or surgical treatment, to assist the rehabilitation of vocal and swallowing functions.

Complications. As a laryngeal malignancy progresses, dysphagia and respiratory interference may result. When left untreated or advanced, lesions will most likely spread to regional lymph nodes and may further metastasize to other organs of the body. Untreated malignant laryngeal lesions lead to death.

Predisposing factors. Smoking and alcohol abuse are the most often cited factors associated with the development of all laryngeal carcinomas. Some data indicate a role of previous radiotherapy to the neck, dietary deficiencies, and exposure to environmental carcinogenic agents in some cases. Links have also been made between laryngeal cancer and human papilloma virus.

Frequency. Laryngeal lesions (glottic and extraglottic) are reported to be between 2 and 5 percent of all malignancies.

Sex ratio. The ratio of men to women who develop malignant laryngeal lesions (glottic and extraglottic) is 4 to 5 : 1, with the ratio narrowing steadily for the past 20 years.

Familial pattern. Unknown.

Differential diagnosis. Chondrosarcoma, osteosarcoma, salivary gland carcinoma, mucoepidermoid carcinoma, adenocystic carcinoma, and lymphoma.

Classification criteria.

(a) Required for medical diagnosis: Confirmation of malignancy through biopsy and histological analysis, showing abnormal cell invasion of lamina propria or muscle.

(b) Required to attribute a voice problem to the medical diagnosis: Voice disorder not wholly explained by other causes.

Severity criteria
  (AJCC Cancer Staging Manual, 6th edition, 2002).

(a) Medical:

Non-vocal fold laryngeal lesions are staged based on the site of origin—supraglottic or subglottic. Laryngeal anatomic subsites comprised within the supraglottic staging system are false vocal folds, arytenoids, suprahyoid epiglottis, infrahyoid epiglottis, and aryepiglottic folds. The subglottic region is not subdivided.

Supraglottic

T1: Tumor limited to one site of the supraglottis with normal vocal fold mobility.

T2: Tumor invades mucosa of more than one adjacent subsite of the supraglottis or glottis or region outside the supraglottis, without fixation of the larynx.

T3: Tumor limited to larynx with vocal fold fixation or invades any of the following: post-cricoid area, pre-epiglottic tissues, or base of tongue.

T4: Tumor invades through thyroid cartilage or extends into soft tissues of the neck or base of tongue, thyroid, and/or esophagus.

Subglottis:

T1: Tumor limited to the subglottis.

T2: Tumor extends to the vocal folds with normal or impaired vocal fold mobility.

Sex ratio. Puberphonia is typically considered a voice disorder of the young adult male. Some clinicians recognize a form of puberphonia (juvenile resonance disorder) in post-pubescent females.

Familial pattern. Unknown.

Differential diagnosis. An organic etiology (e.g., sulcus vocalis, vocal fold paralysis, endocrine dysfunction) must be ruled out.

Classification criteria.

(a) Required for medical diagnosis: Persistent use of a high-pitched voice in males (or possibly females), typically after having completed pubescent changes, and after other etiologies have been ruled out.

(b) Required to attribute a voice problem to the medical diagnosis: Same as for medical diagnosis.

Severity criteria.

(a) Medical: See Introduction

(b) Vocal: See Introduction

1450. Presbyphonia

Although the vocal changes associated with normal aging described below represent classic characteristics of disordered voice (e.g., pitch, loudness, and endurance changes), some speakers will not consider these changes to be "disordered," but rather, normal consequences of the aging process. Conversely, other individuals will perceive a marked decrease in communicative effectiveness due to voice deterioration associated with aging, termed *presbyphonia*. Individual differences in physical health, communicative environment(s) and demands, and personal resilience may all influence the degree to which normal and abnormal changes in voice affect one's quality of life.

Essential features. This is considered a diagnosis of exclusion and is used to describe the changes in voice production associated with advanced age. Vocal folds may appear thin or bowed in some cases.

Associated features. Changes in voice quality, loudness, and endurance are common. Aspiration, particularly of liquids, may be reported. Hearing loss may contribute to the voice disorder.

Vocal impairment: Persons with presbyphonia complain of a muffled or "thin" voice quality and inadequate volume. Increased breathiness may be perceived. Also, some older individuals complain of a creaky and unstable voice quality.

Aerodynamic characteristics: Possible increase in minimum and average phonatory airflows.

Acoustic characteristics: Variable. Perturbation may be increased and signal-to-noise ratio may be decreased. Reports suggest that fundamental frequency decreases in females and increases in males.

Age at onset. While changes of aging are gradual, data on the aging voice seem to indicate the beginning of these changes after age 65 years.

Course. Literature on the aging voice is divided into the young–old (60–75) and the old–old (76 +); more severe voice changes are found in the old–old population. However, estimates of biologic/physiologic age as correlated with health status may be more predictive of vocal aging than chronological age alone.

Complications. Possible decrease in social or occupational functioning; aspiration, especially of liquids.

Predisposing factors. The underlying factors may include some combination of the following: reduced pliability in the respiratory system, alterations in vocal fold mass/structure and vibratory response (e.g., reduction in muscle bulk, alterations in connective tissue, and alterations in superficial lamina propria, especially in females [possibly secondary to hormonal changes]), cartilage ossification, and reduced joint mobility. Changes in glands and blood supply, as well as neuromuscular control, may also be contributory. Higher pitch noted in older males may be due to muscular atrophy.

Other diseases typical of aging may also contribute to voice change in this population. Complicating respiratory problems such as emphysema, bronchitis, asthma, and other respiratory diseases may have a severe impact on phonatory adequacy.

Frequency. Unknown.

Sex ratio. Over age 65, there are more surviving females than males. Information is not available about the frequency of age-related voice changes across the sexes.

Familial pattern. Unknown.

Differential diagnosis. Neurological or pulmonary disorders, or organic vocal fold pathology not attributable to the aging process.

Classification criteria.

(a) Required for medical diagnosis: Dysphonia (hoarse or weak voice), advanced age, signs of mucosal or muscle atrophy, e.g., bowing or thinness (especially in males); competing diagnoses ruled out.

(b) Required to attribute a voice problem to the medical diagnosis: Same as for medical diagnosis.

Severity criteria.

(a) Medical: See Introduction

(b) Vocal: See Introduction

2000. INFLAMMATORY CONDITIONS OF THE LARYNX

2100. Cricoarytenoid and Cricothyroid Arthritis

Essential features. Reduction of motion in cricoarytenoid or cricothyroid joint, due to inflammation. Palpation of the arytenoid cartilage reveals decreased or no mobility of the cricoarytenoid joint. (Range of motion cannot be determined manually for the cricothyroid joint.) In more severe cases, the arytenoid cartilage or cartilages may become ankylosed.

Associated features. Deep pain localized to the larynx. Arthritis is usually not restricted to the cricoarytenoid or cricothyroid joints, but can involve other synovial joints throughout the body as well. When fixed at midline, dyspnea and stridor may result. Lateral fixation causes weak, breathy phonation, and possible aspiration. The arytenoid cartilage mucosa may be edematous and erythematous.

Vocal impairment. Voice may be weak, breathy. Dyspnea and stridor may occur, depending on location and severity of arthritis. If the cricothyroid joint is involved, pitch range may be reduced.

Aerodynamic characteristics: Variable.

Acoustic characteristics: Variable.

Age at onset. Usually occurs in older adults, but may occur at any age.

Course. Onset of dysphonia associated with arthritis is thought to be gradual and progressive, consistent with primary symptoms of arthritis. Resulting hoarseness may be chronic or intermittent, if time-locked to arthritis flares.

Complications. Possible compromised airway, aspiration.

Predisposing factors. Presence of rheumatoid arthritis in other synovial joints, gout, mumps, tuberculosis, syphilis, gonorrhea, Tietze's syndrome, and systemic lupus erythematosus. Trauma may also result in osteoarthritis.

Frequency. Total number is unknown, however, the larynx is involved in 25% of all patients with rheumatoid arthritis; laryngeal involvement in osteoarthritis is rare.

Sex ratio. Unknown.

Familial pattern. Unknown.

Differential diagnosis. Vocal fold paralysis, paresis, and dislocation must be ruled out by appropriate physical exam (e.g., electromyography for paralysis/paresis; intraoperative arytenoid palpation during microlaryngoscopy, or magnetic resonance imaging to rule out dislocation).

Classification criteria.

(a) Required for medical diagnosis: Reduced range of motion of the joint and associated inflammation; competing diagnoses ruled out.

(b) Required to attribute a voice problem to the medical diagnosis: Medical diagnosis of laryngeal arthritis; local pain on vocalization or swallowing; weak voice, vocal fatigue, not wholly accounted for by other causes.

Severity criteria.

(a) Medical:

Cricoarytenoid arthritis:

Mild: Unilateral reduction in joint range of motion.

Moderate: Unilateral fixation.

Severe: Bilateral reduction in joint range of motion or fixation.

Cricothyroid arthritis: No recognized criteria.

(b) Vocal: See Introduction

2200. Acute Laryngitis

Essential features. Acute laryngitis is a non-specific diagnosis that may be due to a number of etiologic factors, including infectious (bacterial, viral, or fungal) and traumatic (phonotrauma/environmental/reflux) causes. Essential laryngeal findings are evidence of inflammatory response (erythema and edema) and acute onset.

Associated features. Hoarseness is common. Throat pain and cough are frequent. Otalgia may occur. Infection may also involve the sinus, ear, and bronchi, as well as the larynx.

Vocal impairment. Changes in voice quality may include pitch alterations (lower pitch if edema is present, higher pitch if stiffness is predominant), hoarseness, breathiness, and in extreme cases, aphonia.

Aerodynamic characteristics: Variable.

Acoustic characteristics: Variable.

Age at onset. May occur at any age.

Course. Causes may include the infectious (bacterial, viral, fungal), environmental irritants including airborne agents or acute laryngopharyngeal reflux, and/or phonotraumatic behavior. Voice symptoms frequently accompany onset of other symptoms and may resolve either spontaneously or in response to medical and behavioral treatment.

Complications. Persistent dysphonia (Muscle Tension/Adaptive Dysphonia Secondary (8020).

Predisposing factors. Exposure to airborne infectious microbes and/or compromised immune system. Phonotraumatic behaviors are implicated in some cases.

Frequency. Unknown, but common.

Sex ratio. Unknown.

Familial pattern. None.

Differential diagnosis. Bacterial, viral, or fungal laryngitis; acute or chronic systemic disease (e.g., tuberculosis, AIDS, etc.); or trauma (phonotrauma or chemical, environmental, and/or reflux).

Classification Criteria.

(a) Required for medical diagnosis: Evidence of laryngeal inflammation with acute onset; specific cause of acute laryngitis must be established.

(b) Required to attribute a voice problem to the medical diagnosis: Hoarseness, weak voice, vocal fatigue, possibly aphonic breaks and pitch breaks not wholly attributable to other causes.

Severity Criteria:

(a) Medical: See Introduction

(b) Vocal: See Introduction

2300. Laryngopharyngeal Reflux (LPR), Extraesophageal Reflux

Essential features. Mucosal inflammation/irritation due to reflux of gastric contents from the upper esophagus to the pharynx and larynx.

Associated features. Dysphonia, dysphagia, odynophagia, odynophonia, cough, globus, and thickened mucosal secretions. A majority of patients do not report heartburn or gastroesophageal reflux disease.

Vocal impairment. Vocal impairment may range from none to severe depending on severity and chronicity.

Aerodynamic characteristics: Variable.

Acoustics characteristics: Variable.

Age at onset. May occur at any age.

Course. Highly variable; may fluctuate or be progressive.

Complications. Vocal fold granuloma, lung abscess, pulmonary fibrosis, recurrent respiratory disease, aspiration, laryngospasm, apnea, compromised dental or gingival status, halitosis, subglottic stenosis.

Predisposing factors. Gastroesophageal reflux disease, diabetes, obesity, consumption of specific dietary triggers including spicy or acidic foods, dairy products, alcohol, caffeine, peppermints, and many others; tight clothing, exercise, or supine position after eating.

Frequency. Unknown.

Sex ratio. Unknown.

Familial pattern. Unknown.

Differential diagnosis. Gastroesophageal reflux disease, other causes of dysphonia, other inflammatory conditions, infectious processes.

Classification criteria.

(a) Required for medical diagnosis: Positive findings on cephalad probe during 24 hour pH monitoring. In addition, positive response to empiric treatment is commonly used as a diagnostic tool.

(b) Required to attribute a voice problem to the medical diagnosis: Globus, dysphonia, vocal fatigue, or vocal fold lesions not wholly explained by other causes.

Severity criteria.

(a) Medical: One proposed method of stratifying the severity of LPR and possibly determining the presence of the disease is a laryngeal examination scoring system proposed by Belafsky, Postma, and Koufman (2001) called the Reflux Finding Score (RFS). The RFS grades abnormalities and their severity at the following sites: subglottic edema, ventricular obliteration, erythema/hyperemia, vocal fold edema, diffuse laryngeal edema, posterior commissure hypertrophy, granuloma/granulation, and thick endolaryngeal mucus. The authors suggest that an RFS score of greater than 7.0 indicates the presence of laryngopharyngeal reflux and a positive response to treatment with 95 % certainty. In 2002, the same authors proposed the use of a clinical Reflux Symptom Index (RSI), which is a nine-item, self-administered outcome instrument designed to assess the frequency and severity of common symptoms of LPR. Patients rate each item from 0 (No Problem) to 5 (Severe Problem) for symptoms perceived in the last month. The sum of all nine values yields the RSI score; the authors suggest that RSI scores above 13 are considered abnormal.

REFLUX SYMPTOM INDEX (RSI)

Within the last month, how did the following problems affect you?
(0 = No Problem; 5 = Severe Problem)

1. Hoarseness or a problem with your voice	1 2 3 4 5
2. Clearing your throat	1 2 3 4 5
3. Excess throat mucus or postnasal drip	1 2 3 4 5
4. Difficulty swallowing food, liquids, or pills	1 2 3 4 5
5. Coughing after you ate or lying down	1 2 3 4 5
6. Breathing difficulties or choking episodes	1 2 3 4 5
7. Troublesome or annoying cough	1 2 3 4 5
8. Sensations of something sticking in your throat or a lump in your throat	1 2 3 4 5
9. Heartburn, chest pain, indigestion, or stomach acid coming up	1 2 3 4 5

Belafsky, P. C., Postma, G. N., & Kaufman, T. A. (2002). Validity and reliability of the reflux symptom index (RSI). *J Voice* 16(2): 274–7. Reprinted from *Journal of Voice* with permission from The Voice Foundation.

(b) Vocal: See Introduction.

2400. Chemical Sensitivity/Irritable Larynx Syndrome

Essential features. Mucosal and/or sensory afferent abnormality of the larynx following chemical exposure. Irritable Larynx Syndrome (ILS) has been defined by the specific constellation of episodic laryngospasm or dysphonia (globus or chronic cough may or may not be present); tenderness of perilaryngeal muscles, specific chemical stimulus which triggers symptoms, and typically, laryngopharyngeal reflux.

Associated features. Muscle Tension Dysphonia Primary & Muscle Tension/Adaptive Dysphonia Secondary (8010 & 8020), globus sensation, dysphagia, frequent throat clearing, cough, paradoxical vocal fold movement.

Vocal impairment. The degree of vocal impairment can vary greatly and may occur intermittently in response to specific stimuli.

Aerodynamic characteristics: Variable.

Acoustic characteristics: Variable.

Age at onset. Variable; more commonly seen in adults.

Course. Characterized by acute onset with persistence of symptoms across months or years, possibly with resolution or plateau. The condition may be resistant to conservative treatment (e.g., voice therapy alone, or avoidance of chemical triggers alone).

Complications. Structural laryngeal complications related to prolonged or severe exposure to chemicals (e.g., laryngeal stenosis, vocal fold granuloma).

Predisposing factors. Exposure to environmental toxins, laryngopharyngeal reflux disease, viral illness.

Frequency. Unknown.

Sex ratio. Unknown.

Familial pattern. Unknown.

Differential diagnosis. Psychogenic voice disorder, laryngopharyngeal reflux disease, Muscle Tension Dysphonia Primary & Muscle Tension/Adaptive Dysphonia Secondary (8010 & 8020), paradoxical vocal fold movement disorder.

Classification criteria.

(a) Required for medical diagnosis: History of environmental chemical exposure with appropriate physical examination findings.

(b) Required to attribute a voice problem to the medical diagnosis: Episodic hoarseness, weak voice, or vocal fatigue linked to specific environmental chemical exposures, with appropriate physical findings, possibly in conjunction with unusual resistance to conservative treatment (e.g., avoidance of chemical triggers alone or voice work alone).

Severity criteria:

(a) Medical: See Introduction

(b) Vocal: See Introduction

3000. TRAUMA OR INJURY OF THE LARYNX

A large number of factors can produce trauma to the larynx. Classically, the types of trauma are subdivided into (a) mechanical, (b) chemical, and (c) thermal causes. Many traumatic events produce a range of sequelae that are indicated under classifications elsewhere in this manual. Examples include phonogenic mechanical trauma, which may produce edema, inflammation, and granuloma formation. In addition, thermal trauma may produce inflammation initially, and scarring in the long term.

3100. Internal Laryngeal Trauma

3110. Laryngeal Mucosa Trauma (Chemical and Thermal)

Essential features. Acute or chronic mucosal changes due to chemical or thermal exposure. Findings are non-specific and are interpreted within the context of the complete history and physical examination.

Associated features. Acute associated features include dysphonia, odynophonia, odynophagia, dysphagia, cough, and hypersensitivity to either ingested substances or environmental triggers, including respiratory distress due to mucosal injury.

Vocal impairment. The degree of vocal impairment will depend on the degree of injury to the mucosa.

Aerodynamic characteristics: Variable.

Acoustic characteristics: Variable.

Age at onset. May occur at any age.

Course. Initially, inflammatory mucosal changes are seen (erythema, edema, possible hypersensitivity). In some cases, scar formation may be a long-term sequelae.

Complications. Vocal fold scar, laryngeal stenosis, esophageal stenosis, esophageal perforation, bronchial/pulmonary disease, Muscle Tension Dysphonia Primary & Muscle Tension/Adaptive Dysphonia Secondary (8010 & 8020), phonotraumatic lesions, death. In extreme cases of chemical hypersensitivity, physical/social isolation may be required.

Predisposing factors. Inhalation of thermally extreme gases, inhalation of toxins (smoke, chemical fumes), and ingestion of toxic materials (either extremely acidic or basic, e.g., bleach, detergents). Accidental ingestion of toxic materials occurs most commonly in young children; deliberate ingestion has occurred in individuals attempting suicide.

Frequency. Unknown.

Sex ratio. Unknown.

Familial pattern. Unknown.

Differential diagnosis. Other inflammatory conditions of the larynx (Wegener's disease, Laryngopharyngeal Reflux, infectious laryngitis, Irritable Larynx Syndrome).

Classification criteria.

(a) Required for medical diagnosis:

Acute. Laryngeal mucosal inflammatory process in combination with appropriate history.

Chronic. Vocal fold scar and/or hypersensitivity with the appropriate history.

(b) Required to attribute a voice problem to the medical diagnosis: Pitch changes, hoarseness, vocal fatigue, or odynophonia with onset coinciding with appropriate history.

Severity criteria.

(a) Medical: Severity criteria for mucosal injury can be broken down into acute and chronic categories.

Acute
(a) Limited mucosal inflammation

(b) Stridor without airway embarrassment

(c) Airway compromise

Chronic

(a) Limited mucosal scar

(b) Diffuse mucosal scar

(c) Laryngeal and/or esophageal stenosis

(b) Vocal: See Introduction

3120. Intubation/Extubation Injuries

Essential features. Injury to the larynx due to intubation (short- or long-term) or extubation.

Associated features. Visible manifestations of endotracheal tube intubation or extubation trauma are variable, but may include: mucosal ulceration in the posterior commissure of the larynx; granulation tissue formation, usually on the medial surfaces of the vocal processes, or in the posterior commissure; scar formation, including vocal fold web, laryngostenosis, subglottic stenosis, and tracheostenosis; sore throat with or without edema in glottic, supraglottic, subglottic, and retroarytenoid regions; nerve injury.

Vocal impairment. Degree of vocal impairment can vary considerably, ranging from minimal to significant, depending on the nature and degree of the injury.

> *Aerodynamic characteristics:* Variable.
>
> *Acoustic characteristics:* Variable.

Age at onset. Injuries are not specific to age; onset is iatrogenic and can occur at any age in association with an intubation event. Occult injuries may occur from intubation associated with premature birth.

Course. Injuries to the larynx, supra- and/or subglottic regions can occur during placement of the endotracheal tube, during the period of intubation, or during extubation. The initial symptoms are variable, ranging from mild hoarseness or sore throat to severe post-intubation dysphonia that results in chronic dysphonia. Recovery may be spontaneous following removal of endotracheal tube, allowing for tissue healing. In more severe forms, intubation trauma may result in the need for secondary laryngeal surgery to modify post-intubation sequelae (e.g., excision of granulation tissue or resection of web). Occasionally medical treatments such as steroid or antibiotic therapies may assist in resolving laryngeal edema.

Complications. Depending upon the site and extent of intubation trauma, more severe complications can include tissue rupture (e.g., pyriform sinus, esophagus, other mucosal tears) or mechanical dislocation of cartilages at the cricoarytenoid or cricothyroid joints (see 3010). Ankylosis of laryngeal joints, paralysis, or subglottic stenosis are possible sequelae of intubation injury.

Predisposing factors. Most predisposing factors are related to narrow space relationships in the airway, due to small glottis, short or thick neck size, or cervical arthritis that limits neck extension and mobility. Intubation injuries are more common following emergent procedures when the need for airway management overrides the risk of possible intubation trauma. Likelihood of laryngeal injury increases with duration of intubation, increased size of endotracheal tube, increased cuff pressure, and excessive movement of the tube, especially during mechanical ventilation. Finally, presence of local infection increases the potential for post-intubation chondritis or stenosis.

Frequency. Unknown.

Sex Ratio. Unknown.

Familial pattern. Unknown.

Differential diagnosis. Iatrogenic scar, reflux-induced changes to the larynx, and arytenoid dislocation due to other causes.

Classification criteria. Laryngeal injury associated with short- or long-term endotracheal intubation.

Severity criteria.

(a) Medical: See Introduction

(b) Vocal: See Introduction

3130. Arytenoid Dislocation

Essential features. Arytenoid malposition often associated with reduced range of motion, not due to neurogenic or inflammatory causes.
Disparity in height between the vocal processes and impaired mobility
of the vocal fold on the side where the cricoarytenoid joint is affected.

Associated features. In posterior dislocations, the vocal process and
fold are usually higher on the dislocated side. In anterior dislocations,
they are generally lower on the dislocated side. The vocal fold on the
injured side may be immobilized or may move abnormally. Dysphonia
and pain are typical associated features.

Vocal impairment. Similar to impairments seen for paralysis or paresis of the affected tissue. Typical effects include dysphonia, reduced
pitch and dynamic ranges, rapid vocal fatigue, possibly breathiness.
Post-operative or post-traumatic hoarseness that is unusually severe or
does not diminish on schedule as healing of the tissues and reduction of
edema occurs. Limitations in control of airflow, protection of the airway, phonatory power and other laryngeal functions will be noted.

Aerodynamic characteristics: Airflow is likely to be increased.

Acoustic characteristics: Variable. Fundamental frequency and intensity ranges and control are likely to be affected. Poorer closure
results in reduced intensity. Inability to control vocal fold tension
results in reduced frequency and frequency range.

Age at onset. Dislocation may occur following trauma to the larynx, at
any age.

Course. Acute onset of dysphonia typically occurs within two or three
days following trauma to the neck, including external trauma (e.g., motor vehicle accident), extubation, anesthesia, and surgery.

Complications. Often not accurately diagnosed and mistaken for vocal fold paralysis. Restoration of vocal fold function is most effectively achieved if attempted soon after the injury by surgical reduction. Occasionally, the dislocation will result in respiratory obstruction.

Predisposing factors. Mechanical trauma to the larynx. Anatomic factors that result in difficult endotracheal intubation predispose to arytenoid dislocation. The risk of dislocation increases in persons with small larynges who undergo intubation, and with the use of an endotracheal tube that is disproportionately large relative to the size of the larynx.

Frequency. Unknown.

Sex ratio. Unknown.

Familial pattern. None.

Differential diagnosis. Vocal fold paralysis, joint fixation.

Classification criteria.

(a) Required for medical diagnosis: Reduced vocal fold mobility/ arytenoids mal-position not due to neuromuscular factors, or inflammation. Laryngeal electromyography and arytenoid palpation are most helpful for diagnosis. CT scan or magnetic resonance imaging may also be useful to confirm diagnosis.

(b) Required to attribute a voice problem to the medical diagnosis: Weak, hoarse voice not wholly accounted for by other conditions.

Severity criteria.

(a) Medical: For anterior and posterior dislocations, severity is determined by degree of arytenoid mobility.

(b) Vocal: See Introduction

3200. External Laryngeal Trauma

Essential features. Injury or dysfunction of the larynx following trauma to the external laryngeal framework.

Associated features. Depends on position, nature, and severity of trauma. Variable voice and/or airway changes may be present.

Vocal impairment. Variable, depending on position, nature, and severity of trauma.

Aerodynamic characteristics: Variable across individuals.

Acoustic characteristics: Variable across individuals.

Age at onset. Any age.

Course. Sudden onset following trauma. Resolution can occur spontaneously or with medical or behavioral intervention, or deficits can be persistent.

Complications. Laryngotracheal stenosis, fractures, dislocation, and other airway complications may result.

Predisposing factors. Trauma to the larynx. Examples include seatbelt, strangulation, and blunt or open trauma.

Frequency. Unknown.

Sex Ratio. Unknown.

Familial pattern. Unknown.

Differential diagnosis. Internal laryngeal trauma; neuromuscular deficits that may mimic trauma or co-exist with it.

Classification criteria.

(a) Required for medical diagnosis: Anatomic changes to laryngeal framework subsequent to external trauma.

(b) Required to attribute a voice problem to the medical diagnosis:
Voice changes consistent with anatomic findings of physical examination, with appropriate medical history, not wholly attributable to other causes.

Severity criteria.

(a) Medical:

Mild: Soft tissue injury without framework disruption.

Moderate: Laryngeal framework disruption with or without soft tissue injury not requiring surgical intervention.

Severe: Laryngeal framework disruption requiring surgical intervention for significant voice problems and/or airway preservation.

(b) Vocal: See Introduction

4000. SYSTEMIC CONDITIONS AFFECTING VOICE

4100. Endocrine

4110. Hypothyroidism

Essential features. Deficiency in thyroid hormone levels. Prolonged levels of hypothyroidism may result in vocal fold edema.

Associated features. Removal or loss of functioning thyroid tissue results in myxedema. Myxedema is characterized by edema within the subcutaneous tissue (potentially in the larynx or elsewhere), dryness and loss of hair, subnormal body temperature, and hoarseness and muscle weakness. Infantile myxedema begins during infancy as a result of some acquired injury or disease of the thyroid gland. Congenital atrophy or absence of the thyroid gland results in cretinism, which is dwarfism with intellectual impairment.

Vocal impairment. Hypothyroidism affects the fluid content of the lamina propria causing increased bulk and mass of the vocal folds. These changes cause hoarseness of voice, vocal fatigue, muffled quality, loss of range, and the sensation of a mass in the throat. Findings for voice have not been reported in the literature.

Aerodynamic characteristics: Variable.

Acoustic characteristics: Fundamental frequency may be low.

Age at onset. May occur at any age when thyroid hormone level is absent or depleted. Hypothyroidism is common in the aging female.

Course. The time of onset and amount of thyroid hormone available affect the severity of symptoms and course of the disorder. In adults, symptoms may take years to develop. Early treatment to supplement thyroid hormones pharmacologically ameliorates symptoms in general, although vocal symptoms may persist without a known connection to hormone levels. Adult onset does not affect an individual's growth and development to the same extent as congenital or infantile hypothyroidism. Hashimoto's thyroiditis is an inflammatory disease of the thyroid gland, characterized by hyperthyroidism in the early stages, and hypothyroidism in late stages.

Complications. Fatigue and elevated levels of thyroid-stimulating hormones may occur even with low–normal thyroid function. Mild hypothyroidism, as well as myxedema (resulting from severe hypothyroidism), may cause vocal symptoms. Thyroid hormone levels may be difficult to adjust with medication and take time to stabilize. In severe forms, ataxic dysarthria may be noted.

Predisposing factors. Low levels of iodine in the diet.

Frequency. The addition of iodine to salt and improved identification of hypothyroidism in infancy has resulted in a marked decrease in cretinism. Hypothyroidism as a cause of laryngeal changes and voice problems may be under-recognized.

Sex ratio. Unknown.

Familial pattern. Historically, common in Midwest regions due to dietary iodine deficiency.

Differential diagnosis. Laryngeal edema or tissue changes due to other causes (e.g., phonotrauma).

Classification criteria.

(a) Required for medical diagnosis: Laryngeal edema or tissue changes not attributable to other causes in the presence of diagnosed hypothyroidism.

(b) Required to attribute a voice problem to the medical diagnosis: Hoarse, weak voice not wholly attributable to other causes.

Severity criteria.

(a) Medical: See Introduction

(b) Vocal: See Introduction

4120. Hyperthyroidism

Essential features. Elevated levels of thyroid hormone.

Associated features. Prominent eyeballs (exopthalmus), goiter, dysphonia, tremor, tachycardia, unexplained weight loss, and irritability may occur in association with this disease (Basedow's, Flajani's, Graves', Marsh's, Parry's, or Parson's disease).

Vocal impairment. Breathy or tremulous voice quality and reduced loudness may be present.

Aerodynamic characteristics: Variable.

Acoustic characteristics: Variable.

Age at onset. Adult.

Course. Thyrotoxicosis may develop slowly as the thyroxin levels build. Accurate diagnosis may be delayed if problems are attributed to other causes. Hashimoto's thyroiditis is an inflammatory disease of the thyroid gland, characterized by hyperthyroidism in the early stages, and hypothyroidism in late stages.

Complications. Pharmacological treatment may reduce symptoms, but thyroid hormone levels may be difficult to adjust to appropriate levels and take time to stabilize.

Predisposing factors. Unknown.

Frequency. Unknown.

Sex ratio. More frequent in women.

Familial pattern. Unknown.

Differential diagnosis. Vocal fold atrophy, paresis, paralysis, and vocal tremor.

Classification criteria.

(a) Required for medical diagnosis: Voice abnormality associated with elevated thyroid hormone level, not attributable to other causes.

(b) Required to attribute a voice problem to the medical diagnosis: Weak, breathy, or tremulous voice not attributable to other causes.

Severity criteria.

(a) Medical: See Introduction

(b) Vocal: See Introduction

4130. Sexual Hormone Imbalances

Essential features. Imbalances in sex hormone levels, associated with menstruation (laryngopathia premenstrualis), pregnancy (laryngopathia gravidarum), menopause (hypoestrogenic voice changes), or androgen use (e.g., birth control pills).

Associated features. In addition to voice changes, hirsutism (hairiness), gynecomastia (enlarged breasts), and other secondary sex changes may occur or fail to occur.

Vocal impairment. Vocal symptoms related to endocrine changes are idiosyncratic. Generally, premenstrual changes include loss of highest range of fundamental frequency, increased vocal fatigue, mild hoarseness, and other slight quality deviations. Androgens, especially testosterone found in oral contraceptives and medications for endometriosis, may significantly reduce pitch and may affect voice quality.

Aerodynamic characteristics: Variable.

Acoustic characteristics: Variable.

Age at onset. Changes occur in women's voices most frequently during the premenstrual cycle, during pregnancy, and in association with menopause and pharmacological (hormonal) treatments.

Course. Dependent on hormone(s) involved, their levels, and duration of hormonal treatments.

Complications. Deleterious changes in voice quality and pitch may be irreversible due to androgenic hormonal treatments.

Predisposing factors. In addition to the sex glands, other glands such as the thyroid, parathyroid, adrenal, pineal, and pituitary may cause endocrine disturbances that alter the voice. Medications such as ovulation inhibitors, oral contraceptives, estrogen replacements, and androgens are also implicated. Hyperbolic steroids masculinize the voice, thymic abnormalities result in feminization of the voice, and pancreatic dysfunction may result in dry voice (xerophonia). Sensitivity to hormonal fluctuations is inconsistent across individuals. Subtle changes may be more apparent in the professional voice user population.

Frequency. Unknown, but reported more often by singers.

Sex ratio. Appears to occur more in women, presumably due to fluctuations in sex hormone levels.

Familial pattern. Unknown.

Differential diagnosis. Voice changes unattributable to other causes.

Classification criteria.

(a) Required for medical diagnosis: Hormone level abnormality based on tests of thyroid function, dedydroepiandrosterone (DHEAS), androstenedione, cortisol, testosterone (total and free), estrogen, prolactin, 17-hydroxyprogesterone, or relevant agents, as determined by an endocrinologist, excluding other causes.

(b) Required to attribute a voice problem to the medical diagnosis: Changes in vocal pitch, quality, or endurance consistent with hormonal profile, not wholly attributable to other causes.

Severity criteria.

(a) Medical: See Introduction

(b) Vocal: See Introduction

4140. Growth Hormone Abnormalities (Hyperpituitarism)

Essential features. Abnormal enlargement of bone, cartilage, and soft tissue known as acromegaly, caused by excessive secretions of the pituitary growth hormone, somatotropin.

Associated features. Gigantism, Dysphonia, Dysarthria.

Vocal impairment. Voice abnormalities may occur as a consequence of untimely and excessive enlargement of the vocal folds and laryngeal cartilages. Enlarged oral and pharyngeal cavities and increased size of mandible and tongue affect resonance and articulation. Abnormally low pitch, hoarseness, and articulation defects are common.

Aerodynamic characteristics: Variable.

Acoustic characteristics: Variable.

Age at onset. Hyperpituitarism occurs in adults if a tumor in the region of the pituitary gland results in excessive production of the growth hormone. Hyperpituitarism may occur in children who have not yet undergone epiphyseal fusion.

Course. Course is dependent on the timing, degree, and duration of growth hormone secretion.

Complications. Orthodontia may be necessary to help correct mandibular and dental problems associated with this disorder. Psychosocial issues, such as low self-esteem and disturbed peer interactions are noted. Vocational options may be restricted.

Predisposing factors. Usually spontaneous. May be associated with a tumor in the hypophysis.

Frequency. Pituitary tumors are found in 25% of exploratory post-mortem biopsies. However, clinically, the condition is much rarer. One to seven instances are found per 100,000 cases in neurosurgical series.

Sex ratio. Equal, in autopsy series. Clinically, ratio appears slightly higher in women.

Familial pattern. Unknown.

Differential diagnosis. Hyperpituitarism can be either primary (i.e., a neoplasm of the pituitary gland), usually benign (adenoma), or secondary, due to growth hormone secretion by a non-pituitary neoplasm (carcinoid tumor).

Classification criteria.

(a) Required for medical diagnosis: Voice problem associated with abnormal levels of somatotropin in laboratory tests. Clinical examination indicating exuberant structural growth throughout the body, and in the larynx in particular.

(b) Required to attribute a voice problem to the medical diagnosis: Low pitch, hoarseness, and articulation abnormalities not wholly attributable to other causes.

Severity criteria.

(a) Medical: See Introduction

(b) Vocal: See Introduction

4200. Immunologic

4210. Allergic Diseases of the Upper Respiratory Tract

Essential features. Mucosal changes secondary to abnormal release of histamine caused by a specific trigger.

Associated features. Sequelae may include edema, inflammation, increased secretions, and hypersensitivity; hoarseness and alterations in voice resonance; changes in mucous membranes lining the ears, nose, and throat, and/or upper respiratory tract; coughing, sneezing, soreness, throat clearing, post-nasal drip, pain and or pressure in the ears, headaches, and fatigue.

Vocal impairment. Depending on the severity of the allergic reaction, the patient may experience symptoms ranging from mild edema of the vocal folds, which is barely discernible, to aphonia. Hyponasality commonly occurs with allergies affecting the nasal passages. Allergic otitis media may occur.

Aerodynamic characteristics: Variable.

Acoustic characteristics: Variable.

Age at onset. Usually in childhood, though may occur at any age.

Course. Rapid appearance of symptoms after exposure to the allergen, in susceptible individuals. Course may be perennial, seasonal, or be influenced by geography. Symptoms are usually ameliorated by allergen avoidance or medication. However, life-threatening situations may occur when obstruction of the airway develops associated with anaphylactic shock, subsequent to extreme sensitivity or massive exposure to the trigger.

Complications. Secondary viral or bacterial infections may exacerbate the upper-respiratory tract problems. Patients may become dependent upon bronchodilator aerosols and nebulizers. Antihistamines may cause drowsiness, dryness, and complicated voice problems (e.g., increased subglottic pressure for phonation, increased risk of phonotrauma, or resonance changes). Life-threatening obstruction of the airway may occur associated with anaphylactic shock.

Predisposing factors. Family history and exposure to the allergens.

Frequency. One in every five Americans has some form of allergy. However, the prevalence of allergic response specifically affecting vocal function is not documented.

Sex ratio. Unknown.

Familial pattern. If both parents have allergies, there is a 75% chance that a child will develop them; if only one parent is allergic, there is a 50% chance that a child will be allergic.

Differential diagnosis. Infectious causes, laryngopharyngeal reflux disease, post vagal viral neuropathy. Contribution of voice use patterns such as those producing phonotrauma, Muscle Tension Dysphonia Primary, or Muscle Tension/Adaptive Dysphonia Secondary (8010; 8020); medications causing laryngeal drying.

Classification criteria.

(a) Required for medical diagnosis: Accurate and thorough history taking including assessment of present symptoms, diet, medications, seasonal and environmental patterns together with a physician's examination, is essential. Skin testing and/or a radioallergosorbent blood test (RAST) may be used. Trial medical therapy may be used as a diagnostic tool.

(b) Required to attribute a voice problem to the medical diagnosis: Hoarseness or hyponasality attributable to mucosal changes due to allergic responses.

Severity criteria.

(a) Medical:

Mild: Voice changes that fluctuate due to occasional exposure to allergens, with complete resolution following removal of the allergen.

Moderate: Seasonal voice changes associated with environmental allergens, with return of normal voice after seasonal exposure.

Severe: Persistent voice changes associated with exposure to allergens, with no return to normal voice.

(b) Vocal: See Introduction

4220. HIV and AIDS

Essential features. Immunologic T-cell deficit due to Human Immunodeficiency Viral (HIV) infection. HIV is a sub-group of retroviruses that infects the nervous system and weakens the immune system (T-lymphocytes and monocytes). HIV-positive status is confirmed by the presence of HIV antibodies, whereas Acquired Immunodeficiency Syndrome (AIDS) is diagnosed by a T-lymphocyte count of less than 200.

Associated features. Hoarseness may result from recurrent infections of the upper-respiratory tract, specifically oral and/or laryngeal candidiasis (thrush). Ear infections are especially troublesome in HIV-positive infants and children. More important general associated features include constitutional fever, persistent symptoms of a cold, night sweats, weight loss, cough, and in more advanced stages, depression and dementia.

Vocal impairment. Vocal impairment can range from none to severe. Typically, impairments are due to cold-like symptoms or laryngeal or oral candida.

Aerodynamic characteristics: Variable.

Acoustic characteristics: Variable.

Age at onset. Any age.

Course. Progression of infection may lead to dementia and death.

Complications. Immuno-compromised patients are susceptible to opportunistic laryngeal infections and malignancies, including Kaposi's Sarcoma, Non-Hodgkin's Lymphoma, and squamous cell carcinoma. Progressive deterioration may result in few opportunities for satisfying communication. The progressive nature of the disease results in restricted occupational and social options, psycho-social effects, and depression.

Predisposing factors. Intravenous drug use, unprotected sexual encounters with infected partners, or maternal infection during gestation.

Frequency. 733,000 persons diagnosed with AIDS in the United States; estimated 1–2 million have asymptomatic HIV infection. Worldwide estimates vary.

Sex ratio. Women compose only 16% of AIDS cases in the United States. However, this figure increases to 46% in the world.

Familial pattern. No genetic association known; maternal infection during gestation is known transmission source.

Differential diagnosis. Candidiasis; other chronic infectious diseases.

Classification criteria.

(a) Required for medical diagnosis: T-cell count of less than 200 for AIDS. HIV antibody presence for HIV-positive status.

(b) Required to attribute a voice problem to the medical diagnosis: Voice changes consistent with specific physical findings arising from AIDS/HIV.

Severity criteria.

(a) Medical: See Introduction

(b) Vocal: See Introduction

4230. Chronic Fatigue Syndrome

Essential features. Unexplained, persistent, or recurring fatigue of recent or specific onset; unrelated to persistent exertion; not improved by rest; resulting in significant reduction in pre-morbid occupational, educational, social, or personal activities. There may be a connection to elevated Epstein Barr titers.

Associated features. Additional frequent somatic complaints associated with chronic fatigue syndrome (CFS) include: headache, malaise, night sweats, anxiety, mild low grade fever, myasthenia, myalgia, sleep disturbance, neuropsychiatric symptoms (depression), sensation of poor attention and short-term memory, sore throat, tender neck or axillary nodes, and other somatic complaints. Voice problems may be among such complaints.

Vocal impairment. Not documented. Anecdotally, impairment may involve complaints of mild to moderate dysphonia, extremely rapid and pernicious vocal fatigue, and loss of upper vocal range.

Aerodynamic characteristics: Variable

Acoustic characteristics: Variable.

Age at onset. CFS onset peaks between 25 and 45 years of age.

Course. Symptoms may be exacerbated by physical activity or emotional distress. Symptoms generally worsen over time. In rare cases, symptoms may gradually remit over approximately 3 months. Less than 1/3 of patients have symptom remission after one year. Predictive factors for the persistence of symptoms include age older than 38 at symptom onset, more than 1.5 year history of symptoms, pre-morbid long-term depression, more than eight non-CFS symptoms, which are not explained medically, limited educational background.

Complications. Withdrawal from activities of daily living initially, followed by inability to work. Consequences can include isolation, frustration, anger, and depression.

Predisposing factors. CFS may begin with a viral infection.

Frequency. 2–7.3 per 100,000.

Sex ratio. Twice as many women as men develop CFS.

Familial pattern. Unknown.

Differential diagnosis. Fibromyalgia; Lyme disease; anemia; cancer; hypothyroidism; congestive heart failure; chronic lung disease; chronic liver disease (elevated Epstein Barr titers); chronic renal failure; systematic inflammatory disease; depression; neuropathy; somatoform disorder, psychogenic, or adaptive voice disorder; psychiatric, or other organic causes of symptoms.

Classification criteria.

(a) Required for medical diagnosis: Unexplained, persistent, or recurring fatigue of recent or specific onset; unrelated to persistent exertion; not improved by rest; resulting in significant reduction in pre-morbid occupational, educational, social, or personal activities. Additionally, four of the following symptoms are present or recur for 6 months consecutively, not present pre-morbidly: self-perceived reduction in attention or short-term memory; sore throat; tender neck or axillary nodes; myalgia; multiple joint pain without swelling or redness; headaches; ineffective sleep; weakness following exercise not resolving within 24 hours.

(b) Required to attribute a voice problem to the medical diagnosis: Dysphonia, vocal fatigue, or odynophonia not wholly attributable to other causes.

Severity criteria.

(a) Medical:

Mild: Mild or occasional vocal disruption subsequent to voice use.

Moderate: Moderate or recurring vocal disruption subsequent to voice use.

Severe: Severe or persistent vocal disruption subsequent to voice use.

(b) Vocal: See Introduction

4240. Systemic Lupus Erythematosus

Essential features. Systemic Lupus Erythematosus (SLE) is a chronic rheumatologic disease having antibodies that are directed against self-antigens, immune complex formation, and immune disregulation. More simply, the body loses the ability to distinguish between harmful foreign bodies and endogenous cells and tissues. Thus, the cells of the immune system attack normal cells in the body. This complex circulates and disrupts normal organic functioning, particularly in the kidneys. Affecting voice, lupus complexes may deposit in the esophagus, causing significant reflux and thus laryngeal changes. Laryngeal manifestations of lupus may involve laryngeal ulcerations of the anterior, superior larynx that progress to fibrotic lesions often showing exudate, which may form a scar after healing. Laryngeal lupus is primarily confined to the anterior larynx, involving the epiglottis and the anterior portion of the aryepiglottic folds; the posterior larynx is rarely involved.

Associated features. Laryngopharyngeal reflux; dysphagia; butterfly-shaped rash across the cheeks and nose; possibly yellowish-pink discrete nodule lesions found in the anterior larynx usually occurring in association with the onset of symptoms; Reynaud's syndrome (discoloration of fingers exposed to cold). Lesions are generally painless; patients typically report reduced sensation in the involved areas. Despite anterior laryngeal involvement of lupus lesions, voice quality is not usually involved until later stages.

Vocal impairment.

Aerodynamic characteristics: Variable.

Acoustic characteristics: Variable.

Age at onset. Onset of SLE occurs between 15–45 years for 80% of individuals with the disease.

Course. Lupus is an incurable chronic autoimmune disease. The disease leads to inflammation of various body parts. In advanced stages, the disease can be life-threatening.

Complications. Reflux, dysphagia, vocal fold lesions, kidney failure, and death.

Predisposing factors. Female, Native American, Asian, African-American, Latin-American.

Frequency. Approximately 1.4 million adults have the condition.

Sex ratio. 90% of individuals with SLE are women.

Familial pattern. Only 10% of individuals with SLE have a parent or close relative with the disease.

Differential diagnosis. Other rheumatologic diseases (scleroderma, rheumatoid arthritis, etc.); Chronic Fatigue Syndrome; reflux disease.

Classification criteria.

(a) Required for medical diagnosis: Positive antinuclear antibody (ANA); presence of anti-ANA antibodies.

(b) Required to attribute a voice problem to the medical diagnosis: Voice changes consistent with physical findings (e.g., reflux) or suspected physical conditions (e.g., laryngeal arthritis) associated with the disease. Specific exacerbations of voice problems coincide with flare-ups of the disease.

Severity criteria.

(a) Medical: See Introduction

(b) Vocal: See Introduction

4250. Sjogren's Syndrome

Essential features. This autoimmune disease causes the body's immune system to mistakenly attack the salivary glands. The clinical profile includes xerostomia (dry mouth) and dry eyes.

Associated features. Thick mucous, globus sensation, dry cough, dysphagia, and hoarseness with or without phonotraumatic lesions. The combination of thick mucous and dry surface tissue may result in a thick crusty appearance on surface of the vocal folds. Sicca syndrome is also common.

Vocal impairment. Related to laryngeal dryness, which may increase the risk of phonotraumatic lesions, vocal fatigue, or Muscle Tension/Adaptive Dysphonia (8020).

Aerodynamic characteristics: Variable.

Acoustic characteristics: Variable.

Age at onset. Primarily affects women between ages of 40–50 years.

Course. The course is generally mild and benign. However, complications include the possibility of painful eye irritation, severe dental caries, and painful intercourse (dyspareunia). Because symptoms are often insidious, patients may not seek medical attention until later in the disease course. The disease is incurable.

Complications. A 40% increase in specific types of cancer (lymphoma) has been reported in association with Sjogren's disease.

Predisposing factors. Female. Ethnic groups are similar to those for the United States.

Frequency. An estimated 500,000–2,000,000 individuals have the condition in the United States.

Sex ratio. The ratio is 9:1, female to male.

Familial pattern. Unknown.

Differential diagnosis. Rheumatoid arthritis, systemic lupus; scleroderma; polymyocitis/dermatomyocitis.

Classification criteria.

(a) Required for medical diagnosis: Auto-antigens SSA, SSB, and/or ANA, derived rheumatologic workup; other positive signs may derive from lip biopsy or eye examination.

(b) Required to attribute a voice problem to the medical diagnosis:
Voice changes traceable to laryngeal dryness in the presence of positive medical diagnosis.

Severity criteria.

(a) Medical: See Introduction

(b) Vocal: See Introduction

4260. Scleroderma.

Essential features. This systemic disease involves progressive fibrosis and narrowing of the microvasculature due to exuberant production and deposition of collagen Types I and III. Typical consequences include thickening, tightening, and hardening of the skin of the fingers and hand joints. Changes may involve the entire limb, face, trunk, and neck.

Associated features. Reynaud's syndrome (whitening of the digits with exposure to cold); gastroesophageal reflux; dyspnea; chest pain; cough; arthralgia; myalgia; reduction in joint range of motion; carpal tunnel syndrome; fatigue; weight loss; facial pain; reduction in sensation of the extremities; sicca syndrome including xerostomia.

Vocal impairment. Vocal impairments may be due to deposition of collagen within the lamina propria. In addition, vocal impairment may be due to reflux disease.

Aerodynamic characteristics: Variable.

Acoustic characteristics: Variable.

Age at onset. Peak age of onset is ages 30–40 years.

Course. Ten-year survival rates are roughly 60–70% for patients with limited involvement. This figure reduces dramatically to 20% for 10-year survival rate, for patients with diffuse involvement.

Complications. The most common cause of mortality is pulmonary hypertension and its sequelae.

Predisposing factors. Risk is slightly higher for women of African descent.

Frequency. Estimated incidence is 19 cases per million in the U.S. Prevalence is thought to have increased due to improved diagnosis and increased survival rates.

Sex ratio. Risk is increased 3–8 times for women compared to men.

Familial pattern. Unknown.

Differential diagnosis. Eosinophilia; graft versus host disease; mycosis fungoidosis; primary biliary cirrhosis; primary pulmonary hypertension; reflux sympathetic dystrophy.

Classification criteria.

(a) Required for medical diagnosis: Rheumatologic workup indicating ANA, usually with a speckled homogenous pattern.

(b) Required to attribute a voice problem to the medical diagnosis: Voice complaints consistent with physical findings of the disease (e.g., increased phonatory effort found in conjunction with xerostomia; vocal fatigue found in conjunction with arthralgia; laryngeal pain and hoarseness in conjunction with reflux, etc.).

Severity criteria.

(a) Medical: See Introduction

(b) Vocal: See Introduction

4270. Wegener's Disease

Essential features. Autoimmune disease characterized by necrotizing granulomas with vasculitis. Symptoms are most often limited to the upper respiratory tract or kidneys; may also be systemic.

Associated features. Subglottic stenosis due to the granulomatous process, nasal obstruction, neurologic involvement, saddle deformity of the nose due to destruction of the nasal cartilage, conductive hearing loss, voice problems, and/or stridor secondary to subglottic or posterior glottic stenosis and their treatments.

Vocal impairment. Vocal impairment due to Wegener's disease usually follows neural or structural damage to the larynx and its innervation secondary to surgical procedures of the trachea. Vocal fold paralysis is a potential sequelae.

Aerodynamic characteristics: Variable.

Acoustic characteristics: Variable.

Age at onset. Peak onset is in the 4th to 5th decade.

Course. Progressive. As inflammatory process continues to involve the airway, the condition becomes life threatening. Wegener's disease has a mortality rate of 13% at 8 years, with rates as high as 36% at 10 years.

Complications. Poor healing from surgical procedures, especially occurring in the nose and sinuses. Subglottic stenosis may require surgical intervention including dilatations, carbon-dioxide laser resections, and laryngotracheoplasty with or without microvascular reconstruction. At a systemic level, cancer may result from prolonged immunosuppression treatment.

Predisposing factors. Individuals with Wegener's disease are predominantly Caucasian (97%).

Frequency. 1 in every 30,000–50,000 individuals.

Sex ratio. Slightly more common in males.

Familial pattern. Unknown.

Differential diagnosis. Good Pasture Syndrome; lupus; midline granuloma.

Classification criteria.

(a) Required for medical diagnosis: Positive results of C-ANCA (anti-neutrophilic cytoplasmic antibody) test.

(b) Required to attribute a voice problem to the medical diagnosis: Voice changes consistent with the patient's specific physical findings (e.g., hoarseness in conjunction with vocal fold paralysis due to tracheal surgeries).

Severity criteria.

(a) Medical: See Introduction

(b) Vocal: See Introduction

4300. Musculo-Skeletal Conditions Affecting Voice

4310. Overuse Injury and Repetitive Strain Injury (RSI)

RSI is reported to be the fastest growing occupational injury nationwide, accounting for billions of dollars of economic losses to society annually. Although the condition commonly manifests in the digits subsequent to heavy keyboard use, the condition may extend to the larynx when voice recognition software is instituted. Increasingly, individuals with RSI affecting the voice are seen clinically.

Essential features. Tissue damage caused by repetitive motion, rather than by an isolated event or disease. Overuse injuries include a spectrum of conditions, primary among which is Repetitive Strain Injury (RSI). Various arguments are made about the relative connection—or not—of overuse injury and RSI to tendonitis, bursitis, and carpal tunnel syndrome.

Associated features. Pain; occupational and social restriction; depression; frustration with ineffective medical treatment. In RSI, associated features also include sensitivity to cool temperatures, extremely cold extremities even in warm environments, and in advanced cases, difficulty with simple tasks of daily living. Various reports further implicate the causal presence of chronic rheumatic pain syndrome, cervical syndrome, vasodilatation and restricted vaso-motion, and degradation of sensory representations of movement in the cortex, for RSI. RSI may affect voice when digital keyboard users switch to voice recognition systems to control computers and in other scenarios that involve repetitive use of voice (e.g., reception staff, telemarketing, etc.).

Vocal impairment. Vocal impairment in RSI typically involves weak, muted voice, odynophonia, and extremely rapid onset of vocal fatigue.

Aerodynamic characteristics: Unknown.

Acoustic characteristics: Unknown.

Age at onset. Specific figures are not available for the family of over-use injuries in general. However, adolescent and adult onset of RSI are presumed to be more common because of the increase in cumulative tissue use with increased age.

Course. Typically, a gradual onset of symptoms, which worsen with continued limb or digit use. Postural and voice use changes may improve symptoms, if onset is recent (within a few months). Symptoms are more resistant to recovery with longstanding injuries; such improvements may be seen gradually over a 1 to 2-year period. Many individuals with RSI retain some residual symptoms even after significant and prolonged treatments.

Complications. Compromise in occupational, social, and familial functions.

Predisposing factors. For RSI, the primary risk factor is repetitive motion, and common occupational risks include athletics, typing, piano, and other instrument playing. Chronic, posturally-induced narrowing of the thorax is also implicated as a risk factor in RSI.

Frequency. Frequency of RSI (all sources) increased from 20,000 cases reported annually in 1980 to 700,000 cases in 1996. Prevalence of voice related RSI is unknown, though data suggest that select occupations (e.g., teachers, telemarketers, stock traders, etc.) pose the highest risks.

Sex ratio. For RSI, women are disproportionately involved, possibly because of a high occurrence of women in jobs requiring keyboards.

Familial pattern. Unknown.

Differential diagnosis. Bursitis, tendonitis, carpal tunnel syndrome, cervical strain and sprain; neurologic disease (e.g., myasthenia gravis); psychogenic condition.

Classification criteria.

(a) Required for medical diagnosis: History of chronic, repetitive motion of the affected body part, weakness, fatigue, and pain.

(b) Required to attribute a voice problem to the medical diagnosis: Weak voice, odynophonia, rapid vocal fatigue following a history of repetitive strain injury in the limbs, or chronic vocal overuse. Symptoms must not be attributable to other causes.

Severity criteria.

(a) Medical:

Mild: Minimal symptoms which remit within a few weeks of treatment and that cause little or no compromise in occupational, social, or familial function.

Moderate: Moderate symptoms causing reductions in occupational, social, or familial function, that improve following extended treatment.

Severe: Severe symptoms causing wholesale compromise in occupational, social, or familial function, that fail to improve significantly with extended treatment.

(b) Vocal: See Introduction

4320. Fibromyalgia

Essential features. Decreased pain perception threshold due to altered processing of nocioceptive stimuli. Fibromyalgia is a member of a class of syndromes associated with chronic fatigue and pain.

Associated features. Depression, anxiety, dysphonia, weight fluctuations, attention and memory deficits, allergy symptoms, regional pain, shortness of breath, syncope, frequent urgent urination, odynophonia.

Vocal impairment. Most commonly, patients present with odynophonia, weak voice, and rapid onset of vocal fatigue.

Aerodynamic characteristics: Unknown.

Acoustic characteristics: Unknown.

Age at onset. Any age.

Course. Fibromyalgia is thought to be a chronic, relapsing condition.

Complications. Complications are primarily psychosocial (withdrawal from occupational and social activity, depression, prolific seeking of medical intervention).

Predisposing factors. Some combination of the following: genetic disruption of serotonin metabolism, female, poor sleep, poor physical conditioning, sympathetic or autonomic nervous system disregulation, hypotension of neural causes, viruses or other infections, decrease in collagen cross-linking (hypermobility), cognitive behavioral factors (e.g., abusive familial background, reduction in goal oriented behavior, poor mood).

Frequency. 3–5% of adult females; 0.5–1.6% of adult males.

Sex ratio. More common in females (9:1).

Familial pattern. See predisposing factors.

Differential diagnosis. Anxiety disorders, conversion reactions, depression, menstrual disturbance, endometriosis, hypochondriasis, hypothyroidism, insomnia, irritable bowel syndrome, rheumatoid arthritis, sleep apnea, Systemic Lupus Erythematosus; Muscle Tension Disorder (Primary).

Classification criteria.

(a) Required for medical diagnosis: Muscular pain radiating over large parts of the body, fatigue, poor quality of sleep, dolorimetry evaluating pressure pain thresholds at lateral epichondyles and midpoints of the trapezius muscles, less than 4 kg/cm^2.

(b) Required to attribute a voice problem to the medical diagnosis: Odynophonia, voice weakness, and vocal fatigue not wholly attributable to other causes.

Severity criteria.

(a) Medical: See Introduction

(b) Vocal: See Introduction

4330. Ehlers Danlos Syndrome

Essential features. The condition involves a set of more than ten genetic disorders that involve a deficit in the synthesis and structure of collagen and connective tissue in skin, joints, and blood vessels.

Associated features. Hypermobility of joints, fragile skin (easy scarring), tissue hyperextensibility.

Vocal impairment. Vocal impairment may involve rapid onset of vocal fatigue and extreme effort with high pitches attributable to hyperextensibility of vocal fold tissue, which fails to generate normal stiffness during vocal fold elongation.

Aerodynamic characteristics: Unknown.

Acoustic characteristics: Unknown.

Age at onset. Clinical features are recognizable in early childhood. However, diagnosis usually occurs in early adulthood.

Course. Collagen defect is present from birth. However, the condition is manifested clinically later.

Complications. Muscle weakness, difficulty walking in some cases, possibly joint pain and subluxations, easy bruising.

Predisposing factors. Type IV Ehlers Danlos Syndrome, which has been seen in a limited number of cases affecting voice, involves decreased collagen type III.

Frequency. Incidence is about 1 per 400,000 in the population.

Sex ratio. Approximately equal distribution across the sexes.

Familial pattern. The condition is genetically based.

Differential diagnosis. Cutis laxa (loose skin); pseudoxanthoma elasticum (yellowish maculopapular skin lesions; accentuation of skin creases); difficulty with vocal fatigue and upper pitch range due to deconditioning.

Classification criteria.

(a) Required for medical diagnosis: History of long-term hypermobility of joints throughout the body; histology of skin specimens showing disorganized arrangement of dermal collagen fibers with whorled appearance; disregulation in size and orientation of elastic fibers; deficits in collagen fiber striations shown by electron microscopy.

(b) Required to attribute a voice problem to the medical diagnosis: Rapid onset of vocal fatigue and difficulty with high pitches attributable to Ehlers Danlos Syndrome.

Severity criteria.

(a) Medical: See Introduction

(b) Vocal: See Introduction

4400. Dehydration

Essential features. Dehydration is defined as a condition in which loss of fluids from the body, mostly involving water, exceeds fluid intake. In this condition, intracellular fluids are depleted. Fluid loss occurs by way of vapor losses in breathing, and water losses in perspiration, urine, and stool. Together with water, salts are also lost in dehydration.

Associated features. Individuals with dehydration may have increased thirst, dry mouth, or swollen tongue. In advanced cases, weakness, dizziness, heart palpitations, confusion, fainting, and decreased sweating and urination may occur. Urine that is deep yellow or amber may indicate dehydration.

Vocal impairment. Voice may become dysphonic, and increased subglottal pressures may be required for phonation, especially at high pitches.

Aerodynamic characteristics: Variable.

Acoustic characteristics: Variable.

Age at onset. May occur at any age. Infants and the elderly may be particularly vulnerable to dehydration.

Course. Untreated dehydration may advance to dizziness, weakness, heart palpitations, confusion, fainting, decreased sweating and urination, coma, and death.

Complications. See course. The extreme consequence of dehydration is death.

Predisposing factors. Fever, exposure to high temperatures, extensive exercise, vomiting, diarrhea, increased urination, diabetes, difficulty seeking or obtaining safe drinking water (as may occur with infants or disabled individuals, or with certain physical environments), inability to drink due to coma or other health causes, or significant injuries to the skin.

Frequency. Unknown.

Sex ratio. Unknown. Likely balanced across genders.

Familial pattern. Unknown.

Differential diagnosis. Other causes of signs and symptoms.

Classification criteria.

(a) Required for medical diagnosis: Observation of dry skin or mouth, including sicca larynges (inspissated mucous in the vocal tract or on the vocal folds), or dark-colored urine together with history consistent with fluid deprivation or excessive fluid losses, suggest a possible diagnosis of dehydration. Other observations may include fever, increased pulse, decreased blood pressure, rapid breathing, and dizziness upon standing. Degree of dehydration may be quantified by urine specific gravity and presence of ketones in the urine. Increased glucose in urine may point to diabetes, which is a risk factor for dehydration. Also, sodium, potassium, and sugar concentrations as well as BUN and creatine levels may indicate the amount of dehydration and possible causes.

(b) Required to attribute a voice problem to the medical diagnosis: Voice complaints in the presence of thick vocal tract secretions and also in the presence of a history consistent with possible dehydration.

Severity criteria.

(a) Medical: See Introduction

(b) Vocal: See Introduction

5000. NON-LARYNGEAL AERODIGESTIVE DISORDERS AFFECTING VOICE

5100. Respiratory Diseases Affecting Voice

5110. Asthma

Essential features. Asthma is a respiratory disease characterized by increased responsiveness of the tracheal and bronchial lining to various stimuli. The characteristic physiologic response includes airway narrowing, and wheezing on exhalation. Three types of asthma are identified: (a) extrinsic or allergic asthma, caused by an allergic response; (b) intrinsic or non-allergic asthma, caused by recurring bronchial, sinus, tonsillar, or adenoid infections or bronchial hypersensitivity, due to but not limited to exercise or temperature change; and (c) mixed extrinsic (allergic) and intrinsic (non-allergic) asthma. These conditions may interact.

Associated features. Transitory or prolonged episodes of expiratory wheezing, cough, and dyspnea. Hoarseness may result from impaired respiratory function, or vocal fold changes caused by cough or asthma medications.

Vocal impairment. Type and degree of vocal impairment will depend on degree of mucosal inflammation due to coughing or medications. Often, compensatory respiratory or laryngeal responses may complicate the clinical picture.

Aerodynamic characteristics. Variable.

Acoustic characteristics. Variable.

Age at onset. Asthma with childhood onset is often associated with viral exposure. The incidence of asthma in young children has been escalating in recent years and is often associated with allergic sensitivities. Onset may also occur in later years.

Course. The condition is typically chronic, with intermittent exacerbation depending on the presence of triggering stimuli, compliance with treatment, and treatment success. In severe cases, exacerbation may require hospitalization and even mechanical ventilation.

Complications. Disruption in daily life varies across asthmatic patients, depending on the severity of the condition as well as the level of anxiety regarding the airway obstruction. More anxious individuals may require more medication and hospitalizations than stoic individuals regardless of the actual severity of the obstruction. Asthmatic individuals may restrict various physical activities and avoid certain environments for fear of exacerbating symptoms. Severe bronchoconstriction and mucus plugging of airways may result in hypoxemia. The disease is usually not fatal. However, when the respiratory muscles cannot compensate for airway narrowing to maintain alveolar ventilation, hypercapnia and subsequent respiratory failure can occur. The death rate is on the increase in the U.S. (currently 2 deaths per 100,000 in the population).

Predisposing factors. Family or personal history of allergy; cigarette smoke; concomitant bronchiolitis or pneumonia; congestive heart failure; pulmonary embolism; dusty or windy environments; air pollutants; exposure to pets or previously dampened carpets; mold; exposure to cold air or extended exercise, for some individuals; stress; reflux; unidentified allergic factors.

Frequency. Estimates indicate that 14.6 million individuals have asthma in the U.S.

Sex ratio. More common in females than males.

Familial pattern. Epidemiologic and twin studies show that there is a strong, but not exclusive, genetic predisposition to the development of asthma.

Differential diagnosis. Paradoxical Vocal Fold Motion; foreign body or other source of airway obstruction; extra-esophageal reflux; chronic obstructive pulmonary disease; pneumonia; lung cancer.

Classification criteria.

(a) Required for medical diagnosis: Reduction of forced expiratory volume in 1 sec (FEV–1) and reduction in Forced Vital Capacity (FVC) indicate airway obstruction. Spirometry measures are performed before and after inhalation of a bronchodilator to assess reversibility of symptoms. If spirometry measures approximate normal (as in intermittent or exercise-induced forms of disease), a bronchoprovocation with methacholine or histamine may be performed (methacholine challenge test).

(b) Required to attribute a voice problem to the medical diagnosis: Hoarseness, loss of high notes, vocal effort and fatigue consistent with physical findings of asthma or known pharmacologic side effects.

Severity criteria.

(a) Medical: The National Asthma Education and Prevention Program from the National Heart, Lung, and Blood Institute (NHLBI) suggests the following approach to the rating of asthma severity:

> *Step 1—Mild intermittent:* Daytime symptoms two or fewer times per week, nocturnal symptoms two or fewer times per month, PEF or FEV_1 equal to 80% of normal or better, PEF variation less than 20%.

> *Step 2—Mild persistent:* Daytime symptoms 3–6 times per week, nocturnal symptoms 3–4 times per month, PEF or FEV_1 equal to 80% of normal or better, PEF variation 20–30%.

> *Step 3—Moderate persistent:* Daytime symptoms daily, nocturnal symptoms five or more times per month, PEF or FEV_1 equal to 60–80% of normal, PEF variation more than 30%.

> *Step 4—Severe persistent:* Daytime symptoms always, nocturnal symptoms frequently, PEF or FEV_1 less than or equal to 60% of normal, PEF variation more than 30%.

> *PEF = Peak Expiratory Flow

> *FEV_1 = Forced Expiratory Volume (in the first second)

(b) Vocal: See Introduction

5120. Chronic Obstructive Pulmonary Disease

Essential features. Chronic Obstructive Pulmonary Disease (COPD) is a clinical condition associated with a group of diseases characterized by persistent slowing of airflow during expiration. These diseases may include emphysema and chronic bronchitis. Emphysema is characterized by abnormal, permanent enlargement of air spaces distal to the terminal bronchiole, accompanied by the destruction of their walls, and without obvious fibrosis. Chronic bronchitis connotes inflammation of the large bronchi and excess mucus secretion in the bronchial tree. Individually or in combination, these diseases may cause chronic airflow obstruction, which is the primary feature of COPD.

Associated features. May include dyspnea, wheezing, cough, and sputum expectoration. Activities may be limited due to decreased breath supply. Hoarseness may result from impaired respiratory function or vocal fold injury caused by chronic cough or changes in the vocal fold mucous membrane caused by medications.

Vocal impairment. Related to the severity of the airway obstruction, the amount and strength of associated coughing, and the effect of medications that may affect the lining of the vocal folds. Weakness and inadequate volume due to impaired respiratory function are common.

Aerodynamic characteristics. Variable.

Acoustic characteristics. Perturbation values may be increased, and signal-to-noise ratios may be decreased, if laryngeal inflammation is present.

Age at onset. The condition is most common in middle-aged to elderly adults.

Course. COPD has gradual onset and has usually been present in a subclinical stage for several years by the time the patient is first seen by a physician. As the airway obstruction increases over time, the patients' complaints of breathlessness also increase. In terminal stages, patients may experience lassitude, anorexia, sleep disturbances, depression, and weight loss. COPD is life-threatening because of the destruction of the airway exchange component of the respiratory system (alveoli).

Complications. The condition may significantly affect quality of life as patients are often restricted in physical activities due to the chronic airflow obstruction. The extreme complication is death.

Predisposing factors. Cigarette smoking has been implicated as the most common predisposing factor. Other factors include air pollution, airway hyperresponsiveness, and alpha-1 antitrypsin (AAT) deficiency, which is the only known genetic risk factor.

Frequency. Various studies have revealed that 8–25% percent of the general population and about 50% of middle-aged smokers demonstrate some evidence of COPD.

Sex Ratio. Studies suggest that COPD occurs more in men than in women. However, as gender differences in cigarette consumption continue to narrow, gender differences in the frequency of COPD are decreasing.

Familial pattern. Familial clustering of COPD has been noted from clinical observation. AAT deficiency is the only known genetic risk factor.

Differential diagnosis. Asthma; bronchitis; pulmonary foreign body; tracheomalacia, pulmonary effusion.

Classification criteria.

(a) Required for medical diagnosis: Reduction in Forced Expiratory Volume in the first second (FEV–1); hematocrit of more than 52% in males and more than 47% in females indicates the presence of COPD.

(b) Required to attribute a voice problem to the medical diagnosis: Voice changes due to respiratory dysfunction consistent with COPD, coughing, or medications.

Severity criteria.

(a) Medical: The American Thoracic Society (ATS) has recommended staging of COPD severity according to lung function.

Stage I: FEV_1 is equal to or greater than 50% of the predicted value.

Stage II: FEV_1 is 35–49% of the predicted value.

Stage III: FEV_1 is less than 35% of the predicted value.

   *FEV = Forced Expiratory Volume

(b) Vocal: See Introduction

5200. Digastric

5210. Gastroesophageal Reflux Disease

Essential features. Gastroesophageal reflux occurs whenever contents of the stomach intrude into the esophagus. Reflux occurs intermittently in all individuals, especially after meals. Gastroesophageal disease (GERD) occurs when the amount of reflux exceeds normal levels causing symptoms with or without damage to the esophageal lining. GERD is distinguished from laryngopharyngeal reflux (LPR), in which digestive contents spill into the hypopharynx and airway (see Section 2300).

Associated features. Symptoms include heartburn, chest pain.

Vocal impairment. Not relevant (see Laryngopharyngeal Reflux), unless aggravated by excessive cough related to bronchial-esophageal reflexes.

Age at onset. May occur at any age but more commonly diagnosed in adults, middle-aged and older.

Course. Course may be intermittent or chronic.

Complications. Esophageal strictures; Zenker's diverticulum; pneumonia; asthma; interstitial lung fibrosis; Barrett's disease; cancer of the esophagus.

Predisposing factors. Any source of decreased pressure in the lower esophageal sphincter or poor gastric emptying may increase the risk of GERD. Such sources include hiatal hernia, esophageal dysmotility, diabetes, gastric surgery, smoking, coffee, chocolate, mint, acidic foods and drinks (tomatoes, orange juice), alcohol, obesity, stress in some individuals, calcium channel blockers, nitrates, beta blockers, progesterone.

Frequency. Occurrence increases over age 40.

Sex ratio. May be balanced between the sexes but is more frequently diagnosed in males.

Familial pattern. Unknown.

Differential diagnosis. Achalasia (incomplete relaxation of the pharyngoesophageal sphincter); esophageal cancer; esophageal spasm; irritable bowel syndrome; peptic ulcer disease.

Classification criteria.

(a) Required for medical diagnosis: Classification criteria for esophagitis, caused by GERD, are: *Grade I:* erythema; *Grade II:* linear non-confluent erosions; *Grade III:* circular erosions; *Grade IV:* stricture or Barrett's esophagus.

(b) Required to attribute a voice problem to the medical diagnosis: Not applicable.

Severity criteria.

(a) Medical:

Grade I: Esophageal erythema.

Grade II: Linear non-confluent erosions of the esophagus.

Grade III: Circular erosions of the esophagus.

Grade IV: Stricture or Barrett esophagus.

(b) Vocal: Not applicable.

5300. Infectious Diseases of the Aerodigestive Tract Affecting Voice

5305. Laryngotracheobronchitis (Croup)

Essential features. Commonly caused by a viral infection of the lower respiratory tract, although no single specific virus has been clearly associated. Para influenza viruses and many bacterial organisms have been implicated. Inflammation and edema of the mucous membrane of the subglottic larynx with extension into the trachea and bronchi result. Essential features are a characteristic barking cough and varying degrees of respiratory distress.

Associated features. Patient may complain of hoarseness, throat pain, and in more severe cases, shortness of breath. Symptoms of laryngitis and signs of obstructed breathing including stridor, congestion, increased pulse rate, and restlessness. Cyanosis may also be present.

Vocal impairment. Voice quality may be hoarse, breathy, or strained depending on severity. Vocal pitch may be lowered in response to inflammation and edema. Respiratory stridor may accompany cases involving respiratory obstruction.

Aerodynamic characteristics: Variable.

Acoustic characteristics: Variable.

Age at onset. Most common in children between 6 months and 3 years of age. Mean age at onset is 18 months. Croup is the most common cause of stridor in children.

Course. Begins as mild URI (e.g., sore throat, nasal congestion, fever). Usually resolved in 4–7 days. Hoarseness frequently accompanies onset of other symptoms of infection and resolves as inflammation and edema resolve in response to medical treatment. 5–10% of individuals require hospitalization. Recurrence rate is 5%. A secondary bacterial infection leads to more severe symptoms in some patients.

Complications. There is a potential for disease spread. Death is an extreme consequence of croup.

Predisposing factors. Exposure to disease carrying individual or airborne infectious microbes and/or compromised immune system. Croup typically occurs in late fall and early winter seasons.

Frequency. Peak incidence is 50 new cases per 1000 children in the second year of life. Unusual after age 6. Overall incidence/prevalence in US is 15,000–40,000/100,000 population in the pediatric population.

Sex ratio. Male to female ratio is 2:1.

Familial pattern. Unknown.

Differential diagnosis. Foreign body; bacterial tracheitis; diphtheria; epiglottitis; inhalation injury; laryngomalacia; measles; peritonsillar abscess; retropharyngeal abscess; vascular ring (right aortic arch), subglottic hemangioma; stenosis.

Classification criteria.

(a) Required for medical diagnosis: Typically, diagnosis is made based on clinical presentation (e.g., characteristic barking cough and associated history). Radiographic findings may reveal ballooning hypopharynx and narrowing of subglottic airway ("steeple sign").

(b) Required to attribute a voice problem to the medical diagnosis: Hoarseness with appropriate medical history.

Severity criteria.

(a) Medical: See Introduction

(b) Vocal: See Introduction

5310. Pertussis (Whooping cough)

Essential features. An acute contagious infection (vaccine-preventable) of the mucous membranes lining the air passages by the bacterium Bordetella pertussis. Disease is named for paroxysms of coughing followed by a loud "whoop" or inspiratory stridor due to spasmodic contraction of laryngeal structures.

Associated features. Patient may complain of throat pain. Excessive secretion of thick phlegm or mucous (catarrh) by the mucous membrane of the upper respiratory tract is observed. Symptoms may also include mild fever, loss of appetite, and vomiting.

Vocal impairment. Voice quality may be hoarse or breathy. Vocal pitch may be lowered in response to vocal fold inflammation and edema secondary to chronic productive cough.

   Aerodynamic characteristics: Variable.

Acoustic characteristics: Fundamental frequency may be decreased.

Age at onset. 70% of cases are younger than 6 years of age. Adults account for up to 25% of all cases. Infants under 6 months are at greatest risk.

Course. Course is divided into three phases. The catarrhal stage, or Phase 1 (1–2 wks), involves symptoms associated with upper respiratory infection, without characteristic "whooping" cough. Phase 2 involves episodes of paroxysmal coughing as described above. Phase 3 is convalescent, with chronic cough that may last for weeks. The condition is an endemic disease, which occurs in 3- to 5-year cycles, usually between July and October.

Hoarseness frequently accompanies onset of other symptoms of infection and resolves as mucous secretion, inflammation, and edema resolve in response to medical treatment.

Complications. There is potential for disease spread. Bacterial pneumonia is the most frequent complication. Others include seizures, encephalopathy and death. Fatality is 1.3% in infants less than 1 month of age. Premature infants and patients with existing cardiac, pulmonary, neuromuscular or neurologic disease are at high risk of complications.

Predisposing factors. Exposure to disease-carrying individual or airborne infectious microbes and/or compromised immune system.

Frequency. In the U.S., 5000–7000 cases are reported each year.

Sex ratio. Unknown. Some reports suggest it is more common in females.

Familial pattern. Unknown.

Differential diagnosis. Adenoviral respiratory infection; mycoplasmal pneumonia; chlamydial pneumonia (staccato cough); respiratory syncytial virus infection; bronchialitis; persistent rhinorrhea; marked lymphocytosis.

Classification criteria.

(a) Required for medical diagnosis: Presence of bacterium Bordetella pertussis in sputum.

(b) Required to attribute a voice problem to the medical diagnosis:
Hoarseness with appropriate medical history.

Severity criteria.

(a) Medical: See Introduction

(b) Vocal: See Introduction

5315. Diphtheria

Essential features. A currently rare (vaccine-preventable), toxin mediated, acute contagious infection by the bacillus Corynebacterium diphtheriae, which lives exclusively in human mucous membranes and skin. The organism forms a characteristic plaque-like membranous exudate over affected structures.

Associated features. Patient may complain of slight headache, malaise, mild fever, sore throat, and croupy cough. A yellowish-white or gray pseudomembrane may be observed adherent to the tonsils, pharyngeal walls, and less frequently in the nose or larynx. Respiratory obstruction may occur in the laryngeal form of the disease necessitating tracheotomy. Dysphagia may also occur.

Vocal impairment. Voice quality may be hoarse or breathy. Vocal pitch may be lowered in response to vocal fold inflammation and edema secondary to chronic productive cough.

   Aerodynamic characteristics: Variable.

   Acoustic characteristics: Fundamental frequency may be decreased.

Age at onset. In eras prior to vaccine, the disease was most common in children less than 15 years of age. With population vaccine use, the disease more commonly has onset in later age.

Course. Symptom onset is gradual, beginning with fever and sore throat. Membrane formation begins in the pharynx and may expand to tonsils, palate, or larynx. Hoarseness frequently accompanies onset of other symptoms of infection and resolves as mucous secretion, inflammation, and edema abate in response to medical treatment. Airway obstruction and death are extreme consequences.

Complications. There is a potential for disease spread. If untreated by appropriate antitoxin, the disease can lead to fatal complications. Mortality rate, if treatment is not initiated within the first four days, is 28%. If treated on the first day of the disease, mortality remains 1%.

Predisposing factors. Currently, the primary risk factor is lack of vaccination or incomplete vaccination, exposure to disease-carrying individual or airborne infectious microbes, and/or compromised immune system. Epidemics have occurred as recently as 1995 in the former Soviet Union. In non-immunized populations, outbreaks of diphtheria are most common in fall and winter.

Frequency. Currently rare, with episodic outbreaks in unvaccinated regions of the world. 0.001/100,000 population in the U.S.

Sex ratio. Unknown.

Familial pattern. Unknown.

Differential diagnosis. Epiglottitis; herpes simplex virus infection; impetigo; bacterial pharyngitis; Epstein-Barr virus.

Classification criteria.

(a) Required for medical diagnosis: Presence of bacillus Corynebacterium diphtheriae in exudates.

(b) Required to attribute a voice problem to the medical diagnosis: Hoarse or low-pitched voice consistent with physical findings in the larynx.

Severity criteria.

(a) Medical: See Introduction

(b) Vocal: See Introduction

5320. Pneumonia

Essential features. A pulmonary inflammation, possibly with consolidation of lung tissue that may be caused by a variety of bacterial, viral, or chemical agents.

Associated features. Symptoms include chills, high fever, chest pain, and productive cough, purulent and, in severe cases, bloody sputum. Dysphonia may be a sequelae in some cases.

Vocal impairment. Voice quality may be hoarse or breathy. Vocal pitch may be lowered in response to vocal fold inflammation and edema secondary to chronic cough, or raised in response to increased vocal fold stiffness. Voice symptoms may range from mild to severe, depending on erythema and edema present in the larynx.

Aerodynamic characteristics: Variable.

Acoustic characteristics: Fundamental frequency may be decreased with edema, increased with vocal fold stiffness.

Age at onset. May occur at any age.

Course. Course may involve chills, rigor, non-specific symptoms of headache, malaise, nausea, vomiting, and diarrhea. An extreme consequence is death. Hoarseness frequently accompanies onset of other symptoms of infection, and resolves as mucous secretion, inflammation, and edema resolve in response to medical treatment.

Complications. Respiratory failure, septic shock, death. Spread of disease in infectious cases.

Predisposing factors. Exposure to disease-carrying individual or airborne infectious microbes, and/or compromised immune system. Host factors: diabetes, alcoholism, chronic obstructive lung disease, immunosuppression (including HIV+), aspiration, Sickle cell disease.

Frequency. Community-acquired pneumonia (outside the hospital): 170 cases per 100,000 people; 20% result in hospitalization. Frequency of disease varies with age. For individuals less than 44 years, frequency is 94 cases per 100,000. For individuals greater than 65 years, frequency is 280 cases per 100,000. Frequency in hospitalized patients may approach 25%.

Sex ratio. Unknown. Some reports suggest disease is more frequent in males.

Familial pattern. Unknown (although infectious causes may increase familial risk).

Differential diagnosis. Atelectasis (reduced lung volume); bronchiectasis; chronic obstructive pulmonary disease; foreign body aspiration; lung abscess; lung cancer; respiratory failure.

Classification criteria.

(a) Required for medical diagnosis: Most pneumonias are classified by their etiology (organism). Examples are bacterial (e.g. streptococcal), viral, fungal, or chemical. A special case of bacterial pneumonia—aspiration pneumonia—is caused by aspiration. In that case, the typical organisms include gram-negative bacteria and staphylococci.

(b) Required to attribute a voice problem to the medical diagnosis: Hoarseness, low pitch, or loss of high notes consistent with physical findings of the disease.

Severity criteria.

(a) Medical: See Introduction

(b) Vocal: See Introduction

5325. Infectious Sinusitis

Essential features. Inflammation of the paranasal sinuses caused by bacterial or viral infection. Bacteria involved in acute sinusitis are part of normal nasal flora. Disease may be acute or chronic. Consequences include decreased ciliary clearance or obstruction of involved sinus.

Associated features. Sinusitis results in catarrhal (excessive secretion of thick phlegm or mucous) or purulent discharge through the nose, or post-nasal discharge. Patient may complain of headache, dental or facial pain, or nasal obstruction. Denasality may also be present. Voice quality may be affected.

Vocal impairment. Voice may be hoarse. Vocal pitch may be lowered in response to vocal fold inflammation and edema secondary to chronic cough due to post-nasal drip. Voice/speech may be perceived as hyponasal.

Aerodynamic characteristics: Variable.

Acoustic characteristics: Fundamental frequency may be decreased.

Age at onset. All age groups are affected.

Course. Course may be acute, sub-acute, or chronic (see classification criteria). Sinusitis is more common in the fall, winter, and spring than in summer. Hoarseness and resonance changes follow onset of other symptoms of infection, and resolve as mucous secretion, inflammation, and edema resolve in response to medical treatment.

Complications. The most significant complications are infections spreading to the eye and brain, with resultant blindness and/or brain abscess.

Predisposing factors. Allergic disease; nasal polyps; sinonasal anatomical abnormalities; exposure to disease-carrying individual or airborne infectious microbes, and/or compromised immune system.

Frequency. Acute bacterial sinusitis affects 14% of the North American population.

Sex ratio. Balanced between the sexes.

Familial pattern. Unknown.

Differential diagnosis. Allergic rhinitis; vasomotor rhinitis; URI; allergic fungal sinusitis; cystic fibrosis; sinonasal foreign body; sinonasal tumors.

Classification criteria.

(a) Required for medical diagnosis: Sinus cultures confirm diagnosis of infectious sinusitis. Criteria for acute sinusitis is symptom duration < 3 wk; sub-acute sinusitis is progression of symptoms over 21–60 days; chronic sinusitis is symptoms lasting > 60 days. Radiographic studies (including CT scans) may also be of value.

(b) Required to attribute a voice problem to the medical diagnosis: Hoarseness and/or hyponasality consistent with physical findings in the larynx or nasopharynx, traceable to sinusitis.

Severity criteria.

(a) Medical: See Introduction

(b) Vocal: See Introduction

5330. Tuberculosis

Essential features. Tuberculosis is an infectious disease caused by the bacilli Mycobacteria, in particular, Mycobacterium tuberculosis and Mycobacterium bovis. Tuberculosis commonly affects the respiratory system, but may affect the gastrointestinal and genitourinary tracts, bones, joints, nervous system, lymph nodes, and skin. Laryngeal tuberculosis is most often associated with tuberculosis of the lungs. In the larynx, posterior lesions that resemble other types of granuloma have typically been reported. Contemporary evidence, however, suggests that lesions may be localized, possibly ulcerated, and not isolated to the posterior larynx. More diffuse edema and hyperemia without granuloma may also be noted. The true vocal folds appear to be the most common laryngeal site affected, followed by the false vocal folds.

Associated features. A smooth subepithelial granuloma develops along with intraepithelial pemphigus (crops of bullae that appear suddenly and then disappear, leaving pigmented spots). Systemic symptoms may include fever, night sweats, and loss of weight, appetite, and energy. Patients may complain of odynophagia. In laryngeal tuberculosis, voice quality may also be affected.

Vocal impairment. Vocal symptoms of tuberculosis laryngitis include hoarseness and odynophonia. Voice quality may be hoarse, strained, or breathy. Vocal pitch may be lowered in response to vocal fold inflammation and edema.

>   *Aerodynamic characteristics:* Variable.

>   *Acoustic characteristics:* Fundamental frequency may be decreased.

Age at onset. 65% of U.S. cases occurred in adults aged 25–64 years. Onset can occur at any age, or may be congenital.

Course. The disease typically occurs via inhalation of bacteria aerosolized by infected individuals. From the lungs, bacteria may spread through lymph and blood to other organs. The lesions may heal by fibrosis and calcification as the disease moves into an arrested or inactive stage. Reactivation or exacerbation of the disease or re-infection give rise to the chronic progressive form.

Complications. There is potential for disease spread. A complication of laryngeal tuberculosis is posterior glottic stenosis and airway compromise. Approximately 7% of cases newly identified in the U.S. end in mortality.

Predisposing factors. Exposure to disease-carrying individual or airborne infectious microbes, and/or compromised immune system. Infection may also result from drinking contaminated milk from cows infected with the bovine form of tuberculosis.

Frequency. A resurgence of tuberculosis occurred in the U.S. in 1986. In 1998, 18,000 cases were reported to the Center for Disease Control in the U.S. (6.8/100,000 population). An estimated 18 million people in the US are infected. An estimated 20–33% of the world population is infected. Highest frequencies currently occur in Russia, India, Bangladesh, Pakistan, and Tibet. Only a small percentage of infected individuals develop symptoms.

Sex ratio. Most significant at extremes of ages. No gender predisposition is recognized.

Familial pattern. None.

Differential diagnosis. Syphilis, aspergillosis, histoplasmosis, blastomycosis, sarcoidosis, Wegener's disease, aspiration pneumonia.

Classification criteria.

(a) Required for medical diagnosis: Positive response to purified protein derivative skin test. The size and duration of response is more significant for the diagnosis than amount of erythema; sputum culture may also be useful. For confirmation in the larynx, positive biopsy and culture of suspicious lesions.

(b) Required to attribute a voice problem to the medical diagnosis: Hoarseness or other voice changes attributable to physical findings in the larynx due to the disease.

Severity criteria.

(a) Medical: See Introduction

(b) Vocal: See Introduction

5335. Upper Respiratory Infection (URI)

Essential features. URI is an imprecise term used to refer to any kind of infectious disease process involving the nasal passages, sinuses, pharynx, larynx, or bronchi. The cause may be bacterial or viral and is usually not accurately known. The most common causes are influenza virus, rhinovirus, and streptococcal bacteria.

Associated features. Patient may complain of throat pain and cough, rhinorrhea, chills, fever, headache.

Vocal impairment. If the larynx is specifically involved, dysphonia frequently occurs in conjunction with laryngeal edema and erythema. Voice quality may be hoarse, breathy, or strained. See Acute Laryngitis (2200).

Aerodynamic characteristics: Variable.

Acoustic characteristics: Fundamental frequency may be decreased or, less commonly, increased.

Age at onset. Variable. Depends on nature of infectious disease but most occur at any age. In the U.S., it is estimated that children in daycare have an upper respiratory infection approximately every three weeks from 6 months to 2 years of age.

Course. Usually resolves within about 7–10 days, in otherwise healthy individuals. Some forms may be associated with a 24-hour prodrome (mild symptoms initially preceding more severe status). Hoarseness may accompany or follow onset of other symptoms of infection.

Complications. Bacterial sinusitis or otitis media, following a viral URI. More severe consequences can occur in immune-compromised, elderly, and infant individuals. Epiglottitis is a possible complication of URI. Complications of streptococcal URI include rheumatic fever, glomerulonephritis, peritonsilar abscess, and toxic shock syndrome. There is potential for spread of disease to speaking partners and family prior to onset of symptoms (prodrome).

Predisposing factors. Winter increases risk of all forms of URI except enterovirus, which is more common in the summer. Exposure to disease-carrying individual or airborne infectious microbes or mycoids, and/or compromised immune system.

Frequency. Varies depending on disease and season. Some forms are more common in environments where hygiene and living conditions are compromised. In the U.S., 40,000,000 physician office visits are made annually because of pharyngitis.

Sex ratio. Common colds occur more frequently in women, perhaps due to increased contact with children. See sections on epiglottitis and laryngotracheal bronchitis.

Familial pattern. None evident, although disease transmission among family members may be likely due to proximity and frequency of contact.

Differential diagnosis. Non-infectious processes of URI (e.g., laryngopharyngeal reflux disease, Wegener's disease, allergic sinonasal disease).

Classification criteria.

(a) Required for medical diagnosis: Characteristic symptom time-course, and symptom resolution with appropriate medical treatment.

(b) Required to attribute a voice problem to the medical diagnosis: Voice changes consistent with physical findings due to the condition.

Severity criteria.

(a) Medical: See Introduction

(b) Vocal: See Introduction

5340. Acute Epiglottitis

Essential features. Inflammatory process of the epiglottis (free margins and laryngeal surface most affected) due to infection with Hemophilus influenza type B or less frequently, staphylococcus or streptococcus bacteria. The inflammatory process may also involve the other supraglottic structures (e.g., aryepiglottic folds and arytenoids).

Associated features. Early symptoms may include dysphagia, sore throat, dehydration, fever, tachycardia, and/or restlessness. Voice quality is not usually hoarse, but resonance may be disturbed resulting in "hot potato voice." Vocal strength and endurance may be compromised due to respiratory obstruction.

Vocal impairment. Mild vocal impairment most common.

Aerodynamic characteristics: Typically unaffected.

Acoustic characteristics: Typically unaffected.

Age at onset. May occur at any age, but most commonly between the ages of 2 and 6 years.

Course. Symptoms of respiratory obstruction progress rapidly and require immediate medical attention (steroids, possible airway intervention, e.g., intubation or tracheotomy).

Complications. Airway obstruction leading to possible death or anoxic brain injury.

Predisposing factors. Exposure to disease-carrying individual or airborne infectious microbes, and/or compromised immune system.

Frequency. Significant reduction due to the HiB vaccine. Incidence in the US is 0.6 cases per 100,000 population.

Sex ratio. Increased in males.

Familial pattern. None.

Differential diagnosis. Croup, bacterial tracheitis, retropharyngeal abscess, peritonsillar abscess, mononucleosis, measles, laryngomalacia, diphtheria.

Classification criteria.

(a) Required for medical diagnosis: Epiglottic inflammation (with or without supraglottic involvement) with positive culture of Hemophilus influenza type B or streptococcus bacteria.

(b) Required to attribute a voice problem to the medical diagnosis: "Hot potato voice," reduced vocal strength or endurance, consistent with physical findings of the condition.

Severity criteria.

(a) Medical: See Introduction

(b) Vocal: See Introduction

5345. Syphilis

Essential feature. Infection with the treponema pallidum organism (in the larynx, treponema pallidum endemicum). Disease is acquired through intimate contact, exposure to infected blood, or passed from mother to unborn child.

Associated features. The larynx may be affected in some cases, typically during the secondary stage of the disease process. Signs include mucous membrane edema and mucous membrane patches, often involving the epiglottis, that are temporary and disappear with resolution of the disease. Polypoid lesions of epithelial hyperplasia (condyloma), presenting as smooth yellow projections on the epiglottis and interarytenoid tissues and occasionally on the true vocal folds, may also be noted. Gummata, a soft granuloma varying in size from a millimeter to a centimeter or more in diameter, occurs in the tertiary (advanced) stage of the disease. Fibrosis may develop with increased edema resulting in respiratory obstruction.

Vocal impairment. Vocal impairment is variable from mild to severe depending on progress of the disease.

Aerodynamic characteristics. Variable.

Acoustic characteristics. Variable.

Age at onset. May occur at any age but more likely in adults. Peaks at ages 15 through 34 years of age.

Course. Hoarseness arises with symptoms of edema that may progress to gummata development. Fibrosis and respiratory obstruction can occur in advanced stages.

Complications. Central nervous disease involvement of syphilis is called neurosyphilis and involves headaches, dizziness, and mood disturbances.

Predisposing factors. Exposure to disease-carrying individual, infectious microbes, and/or compromised immune system.

Frequency. In the U.S., incidence in 2001 was 2.2/100,000 population.

Sex ratio. Balanced between sexes in pediatric population. In U.S., slightly more prevalent in men.

Familial pattern. None.

Differential diagnosis. Erythema multiform, herpes simplex, leprosy, sarcoidosis, amyloidosis.

Classification Criteria.

(a) Required for medical diagnosis: Positive serology screening: VDRL (Venereal Disease Research Lab), RPR (Rapid Plasma Reagin), FTA–ABS (Fluorescent Treponemal Antibody Absorption), or positive culture.

(b) Required to attribute a voice problem to the medical diagnosis: Voice signs or symptoms consistent with physical findings due to the condition.

Severity criteria.

(a) Medical: See Introduction

(b) Vocal: See Introduction

5350. Sarcoidosis

Essential features. Multi-system granulomatous disease of unknown etiology that can also involve the larynx and airway. Hallmark histology of the lesions is noncaseating epithelioid granuloma. Pale, diffuse edema of supraglottic structures may also be noted.

Associated features. In the larynx, the epiglottis is most commonly involved. Noncaseating submucosal granuloma may produce ulcerations in rare cases. Dyspnea and airway obstruction can arise secondary to diffuse edema and exophytic masses if the lesion is large. In addition to epiglottic involvement, the aryepiglottic folds, arytenoids, and ventricular folds may become involved. The true vocal folds are usually not directly involved. Systemic symptoms include fatigue, anorexia, weight loss, and fever.

Vocal impairment. Vocal impairment is usually mild, but may become moderate depending on progress of the disease.

Aerodynamic characteristics: Variable.

Acoustic characteristics: Variable.

Age at onset. Most likely adulthood, especially in the 2nd–4th decades of life.

Course. In the early stage, brownish nodules surrounded by erythema are noted. Later, these may fuse to form diffuse thickening. Hoarseness arises with symptoms of edema and later granuloma. Respiratory obstruction may occur in advanced stages. Unpredictable course with frequent remissions and recurrent symptoms.

Complications. Airway obstruction can occur due to fibrosis and stenosis. Cranial neuropathies, including vocal fold paralysis, can also occur. Other complications include blindness, meningitis, arthritis, and renal disease.

Predisposing factors. Unknown.

Frequency. Overall prevalence in U.S. is 10–40 cases/100,000 population. Disease varies with race, age, and urban versus rural location. Laryngeal involvement may occur in 1–5% of all patients with sarcoidosis.

Sex ratio. Slight increased risk in females.

Familial pattern. None.

Differential diagnosis. Wegener's disease, tuberculosis, syphilis.

Classification Criteria.

(a) Required for medical diagnosis: Diagnosis is made by exclusion primarily. Hallmark is noncaseating epithelioid granuloma. However, since this may occur in other pathologies, it is not definitive. Serology for serum angiotension-converting enzyme can be helpful in the diagnosis and disease monitoring.

(b) Required to attribute a voice problem to the medical diagnosis: Shortness of breath in speech, or other signs and symptoms consistent with physical findings associated with the condition.

Severity criteria.

(a) Medical: See Introduction

(b) Vocal: See Introduction

5355. Scleroma of the Larynx (Klebsiella Rhinoscleromatis)

Essential features. Indurated, circumscribed area of granulation tissue in mucous membrane or skin due to infection with Klebsiella rhinoscleromatis (von Frisch bacillus). Usually affects nose, but can affect larynx or other structures of respiratory tract.

Associated features. Hoarseness and cough occur with scleroma development (e.g., thickening of mucosa with inflammatory exudate). Increasing dyspnea may be observed in advanced cases.

Vocal impairment. Vocal impairment is typically mild, but can deteriorate significantly.

Aerodynamic characteristics: Variable.

Acoustic characteristics: Variable.

Age at onset. Unknown.

Course. Hoarseness and cough arise with scleroma development during early stages. Dyspnea may develop as symptoms become more severe.

Complications. There is potential for disease spread.

Predisposing factors. Exposure to disease-carrying individual or airborne infectious microbes, and/or compromised immune system.

Frequency. Very rare in the U.S. More common in Eastern Europe, Southern Asia, India, Indonesia, tropical Africa, and Latin America.

Sex ratio. Affects females more than males.

Familial pattern. Unknown.

Differential diagnosis. Wegener's Disease, URI, vocal fold granuloma, tuberculosis, actinomycosis, leprosy, syphilis, verrucous carcinoma.

Classification criteria.

(a) Required for medical diagnosis: Positive culture for etiologic agent, gram negative coccobacillus K rhinoscleromatis. The Mikulicz cell is specific to the lesion, and is identified by special stains or immunological fluorescence techniques.

(b) Required to attribute a voice problem to the medical diagnosis: Dyspnea or voice changes consistent with physical findings of the disease.

Severity criteria.

(a) Medical: See Introduction

(b) Vocal: See Introduction

5360. Leprosy

Essential features. Laryngeal leprosy is caused by Mycobacterium leprae or Hansen's bacillus. The larynx is typically affected when infection elsewhere extends to it. Inflammatory nodules that produce scarring are characteristic of the disease.

Associated features. Skin lesions, peripheral nerve involvement with anesthesia, muscle weakness, and paralysis. Hoarseness may be due to nodular infiltration of the supraglottis or vocal folds.

Vocal impairment. Vocal impairment may range from mild to severe dependent upon disease involvement.

Aerodynamic characteristics: Variable.

Acoustic characteristics: Variable.

Age at onset. May occur at any age, but more common in children under age 10, and rare over age 40 years.

Course. Incubation period is variable, typically from 2–5 years or more. Symptom onset is gradual. Initial symptoms may be very mild and disease may go undiagnosed for long periods. Following the initial phase of nodular infiltration, resolution of the disease can result in fibrosis of the previously infected region(s).

Complications. Skin and peripheral nerve involvement can lead to loss of sensory and motor function, particularly in the upper extremities.

Predisposing factors. Exposure to disease-carrying individual or airborne infectious microbes.

Frequency. In the U.S., 150–300 new cases are diagnosed per year and in 90% of those cases, the patient has a history of having lived in foreign countries. Worldwide, the number of new cases detected in 1999 was 13.3/100,000 with the highest incidence in India, Bangladesh, Indonesia, and Myanmar (formerly Burma).

Sex ratio. 1.5–2 to 1 male to female ratio.

Familial pattern. Unknown.

Differential diagnosis. Tuberculosis, syphilis, Wegener's granulomatosis, rhinoscleroma, and neurofibroma.

Classification criteria.

(a) Required for medical diagnosis: Skin smears of suspicious lesions and/or cultures. Serology tests can also be used for diagnosis. Skin and nerve biopsies may aid in diagnosis.

(b) Required to attribute a voice problem to the medical diagnosis: Voice signs and symptoms consistent with physical findings of the disease.

Severity criteria.

(a) Medical: See Introduction

(b) Vocal: See Introduction

5365. Actinomycosis

Essential features. Subacute or chronic infection by actinomycosis bacterial species. Three basic clinical types are distinguished: cervicofacial ("lumpy jaw"), thoracic, and abdominal.

Associated features. Of greatest interest for voice, cervicofacial actinomycosis is the most common type of actinomycosis. The larynx is rarely directly involved. However, localized areas of inflammation with yellow subepithelial granules can occur. Hoarseness, throat pain, and laryngeal edema can occur.

Vocal impairment. Voice quality may be hoarse, strained, or breathy. Vocal impairment can vary significantly depending on disease involvement.

Aerodynamic characteristics: Unknown.

Acoustic characteristics: Unknown.

Age at onset. Any age; peak onset in adulthood (20–50 years of age).

Course. Symptoms begin as hoarseness and/or cough and increase in severity as physical symptoms progress.

Complications. With regard to the larynx, there are no significant complications.

Predisposing factors. History of dental or oral surgery.

Frequency. Rare.

Sex ratio. 3:1 male to female ratio.

Familial pattern. Unknown.

Differential diagnosis. Blastomycosis, tuberculosis, candidiasis.

Classification criteria.

(a) Required for medical diagnosis: Direct identification of organisms on biopsy or culture.

(b) Required to attribute a voice problem to the medical diagnosis: Vocal signs or symptoms related to physical findings of the disease.

Severity criteria.

(a) Medical: See Introduction

(b) Vocal: See Introduction

5400. Mycotic (Fungal) Infections of the Larynx

5410. Blastomycosis

Essential features. Infection by Blastomyces dermatitides.

Associated features. Diffuse nodular infiltration of the larynx and marked epithelial hyperplasia, which may result in vocal fold fixation, ulcer, and/or stenosis.

Vocal Impairment. Severity of vocal impairment will vary dependent upon severity of laryngeal lesions as well as resultant vocal fold fixation. Mild hoarseness and cough may be early presenting symptoms. As laryngeal motility decreases with increased severity of disease process, hoarseness becomes severe; additional symptoms of cough, dysphagia and dyspnea may be present.

Aerodynamic characteristics: Variable.

Acoustic characteristics: Variable.

Age at onset. More common in adults, but may occur as early as infancy. Peak onset is 35 years of age.

Course. Early physical symptoms include inflamed, granular laryngeal mucosa in the early stages, followed by dyspnea, hoarseness, cough, and dysphagia in later stages. Tiny miliary (< 2 mm in diameter) nodules may develop on the vocal folds. Symptoms typically lessen and resolve with appropriate medical treatment.

Complications. Pneumonia and Acquired Respiratory Distress Syndrome (ARDS).

Predisposing factors. Exposure to disease-carrying individuals or airborne infectious microbes. Patients with suppressed immune system, such as those on chemotherapy, etc.

Frequency. Endemic in central and southeastern regions of the U.S. (Mississippi River, Ohio River, and Great Lakes). Within the endemic regions, annual incidence rate of 40 per 100,000 is reported. There are few incidence reports outside of the U.S.

Sex ratio. Unclear; possibly slight male predominance.

Familial pattern. Unknown.

Differential diagnosis. Aspergillosis, Cryptococcosis, Tuberculosis, Histoplasmosis. Type and degree of vocal symptoms are not sufficiently unique to be useful in differential diagnosis.

Classification criteria.

(a) Required for medical diagnosis: Positive culture from sputum collection or biopsy.

(b) Required to attribute a voice problem to the medical diagnosis: Vocal signs and symptoms consistent with physical findings of the disease.

Severity criteria.

(a) Medical: See Introduction

(b) Vocal: See Introduction

5420. Histoplasmosis

Essential features. Infection by Histoplasma capsulatum.

Associated features. May resemble tuberculosis and may produce fever, anemia, enlargement of the spleen and liver, leukopenia, pulmonary involvement, adrenal necrosis, and ulcers of the gastrointestinal tract. Laryngeal lesions are characterized as being tumor-like. The nodular mass is typically brown and can produce ulceration.

Vocal Impairment. Hoarseness, strained quality, severe breathiness approaching aphonia. Severity of vocal impairment will vary dependent upon the degree of laryngeal involvement.

Aerodynamic characteristics: Variable. Severe breathiness to aphonia in the presence of significant lesion.

Acoustic characteristics: Variable

Age at onset. Any age.

Course. Symptoms begin as hoarseness and/or cough, and throat pain. Early physical symptoms include inflamed, granular laryngeal mucosa in the early stages. Symptoms may improve with appropriate and timely medical intervention. In its most severe forms, it can be fatal.

Complications. CNS invasion, death.

Predisposing factors. Living in endemic regions. Immune deficiency also increases risk of infection.

Frequency. In endemic areas, 250,000 individuals are infected annually. Internationally, the fungus is most commonly found in North and Central America.

Sex ratio. 4:1 male to female ratio.

Familial pattern. None.

Differential diagnosis. Blastomycosis, aspergillosis, coccidioidomycosis, mycoplasma infections, sarcoidosis, tuberculosis. Vocal symptoms are not sufficiently unique to be useful in differential diagnosis.

Classification criteria.

(a) Required for medical diagnosis: Positive culture for histoplasmosis.

(b) Required to attribute a voice problem to the medical diagnosis: Vocal signs and symptoms consistent with physical findings of the disease, not wholly attributable to other causes.

Severity criteria.

(a) Medical: See Introduction

(b) Vocal: See Introduction

5430. Candidiasis

Essential features. Infection by Candida albicans, which is a yeast-like fungus. Different subtypes include cutaneous, mucocutaneous, gastrointestinal, respiratory, genitourinary, hepatosplenic, and systemic candidiasis.

Associated features. In the larynx, physical examination reveals white patches on a bright red inflamed mucosa affecting the larynx. Associated signs and symptoms include cough, throat pain, and laryngeal edema.

Vocal impairment. Voice quality may be hoarse, strained, or breathy. Vocal impairment varies dependent upon the degree of laryngeal involvement and severity ranges from mild dysphonia to aphonia.

Aerodynamic characteristics: Variable.

Acoustic characteristics: Variable.

Age at onset. Candidal colonization peaks in infancy and in the elderly (above 65 years of age). Also, mucocutaneous candidiasis is most common in infants and elderly.

Course. When affecting the larynx, symptoms of candidiasis, including oropharyngeal pain, dysphagia, and hoarseness, may resolve spontaneously or require topical or systemic treatment.

Complications. With regard to laryngeal involvement, there are no significant long-term complications. Complications of systemic disease are well-documented.

Predisposing factors. Immunocompromised status (status post chemotherapy, steroid use, and HIV), disruption of normal bacterial flora due to broad spectrum antibiotic use or other factors.

Frequency. Common.

Sex ratio. Unknown.

Familial pattern. Unknown.

Differential diagnosis. Histoplasmosis, Cryptococcosis, Herpes Simplex, Laryngopharyngeal Reflux Disease, Mucositis associated with radiation therapy, Blastomycosis. Vocal symptoms are not sufficiently unique to aid in differential diagnosis.

Classification criteria.

(a) Required for medical diagnosis: In the larynx, the diagnosis is usually made by visual inspection (white patches on bright red, inflamed substrate) with appropriate history. Further information can be obtained from scrapings or smears with supporting microscopic findings of candida morphology.

(b) Required to attribute a voice problem to the medical diagnosis: Hoarseness, phonatory effort, loss of high notes, or aphonia, consistent with laryngeal findings and not wholly attributable to other causes.

Severity criteria.

(a) Medical: See Introduction

(b) Vocal: See Introduction

5440. Coccidioidomycosis
   (Valley Fever, Desert Fever, San Joaquin Fever)

Essential features. Infection by coccidioides immitis. May be pulmonary (most common form), cutaneous, or affecting the brain (intracranial).

Associated features. Associated features are specific to the organs affected. In the larynx, physical examination reveals lesions consisting of nodular masses of granulomatous tissue and laryngeal edema. Symptoms may include throat pain and generalized fatigue.

Vocal impairment. May include hoarseness, strained quality, or breathiness.
   Aerodynamic characteristics: Variable.
   Acoustic characteristics: Variable.

Age at onset. Any age, but more common in adults.

Course. In the larynx, symptoms begin as hoarseness and/or cough and increase in severity as physical symptoms progress. Improvement requires medical intervention.

Complications. Respiratory form is rarely fatal (0.2% of cases).

Predisposing factors. Environment. More serious forms are seen in Hispanic and non-White populations, even when other demographic factors are controlled.

Frequency. Unknown.

Sex ratio. Not described.

Familial pattern. Unknown.

Differential diagnosis. Blastomycosis; histoplasmosis; tuberculosis; Wegener's disease. Vocal symptoms are not sufficiently unique to aid in differential diagnosis.

Classification criteria.

(a) Required for medical diagnosis: Isolation of fungus from sputum, smears, or tissue biopsy. Serologic testing can also be used for diagnostic purposes.

(b) Required to attribute a voice problem to the medical diagnosis: Hoarseness, throat pain, and generalized fatigue, not wholly attributable to other causes.

Severity criteria.

(a) Medical: See Introduction

(b) Vocal: See Introduction

6000. PSYCHIATRIC AND PSYCHOLOGICAL DISORDERS AFFECTING VOICE

This section describes voice disorders that have the primary etiologic characteristic related to identifiable psychiatric or psychological conditions in the patient. Such disorders do not necessarily involve laryngeal tissue changes, although exceptions exist.

Similar to most other medical conditions, psychiatric and psychological disorders affecting voice are not only diagnoses of exclusion. Rather, specific inclusion and exclusion criteria must be met. Information for this section is derived from the *Diagnostic and Statistical Manual of Mental Disorders-IV (DSM-IV)* and other sources (e.g., Roy, Bless, & Heisey, 2000a; Roy, Bless, & Heisey, 2000b). The conditions described in this section of the manual are representative, but not exhaustive of psychogenic conditions that may affect voice. Information is presented to enhance clinicians' understanding of the conditions, and to identify patients for appropriate referral to psychiatric and psychological services.

Accurate differentiation of psychogenic conditions—and their relation to voice—is essential to correct diagnosis, treatment, and prognosis of voice conditions arising partly or wholly as manifestations of psychiatric disease. A special caution is that in patients with known psychiatric conditions, special care must be used to rule out other medical conditions that may contribute to a voice problem.

Some patients present with voice disorders that appear to have a psychogenic component, but do not meet DSM-IV criteria for a psychological or psychiatric disorder. Please refer to Voice Disorder—Undiagnosed or Not Otherwise Specified (9000). This category is appropriate for those patients whose psychological factors do not satisfy the DSM-IV classification criteria described in this section, or for whom the psychological or psychiatric diagnosis is pending.

6010. Somatoform Disorders

Somatoform Disorders encompass an array of conditions including Somatization Disorder (historically hysteria or Briquet's syndrome), Undifferentiated Somatoform Disorder, Conversion Disorder, Pain Disorder, Hypochondriasis, Body Dysmorphic Disorder, and Somatoform Disorder Not Otherwise Specified. Of these, Somatization Disorder, Conversion Disorder, Pain Disorder, and Hypochondriasis are probably the most common to present in voice clinics. Accordingly, these conditions are discussed in this section.

6011. Somatization Disorder

Essential features. History of significant, multiform, physical complaints that cannot be fully explained by a medical condition or substance use. Onset must be prior to age 30, and continue over several years. Complaints are associated with medical treatment or significant alteration in social, occupational, or other functions. Additional criteria include complaints in the following domains since onset: four pain symptoms; two gastrointestinal symptoms; one sexual symptom; one pseudoneurological symptom.

Associated features. A possible complaint for voice is odynophonia and vocal fatigue.

Vocal impairment.

Aerodynamic characteristics: Variable.

Acoustic characteristics: Variable.

Age at onset. Prior to age 30 years. Symptoms are frequently seen during adolescence.

Course. Pattern of recurring symptoms.

Complications. Social, affective, occupational.

Predisposing factors. Unknown.

Prevalence. Somatization disorder estimates range from 0.2% for females, and less than 0.2% in males.

Sex ratio. More common in females.

Familial pattern. Women with Somatization Disorder have 10–20% of first-degree relatives with the condition. Both genetic and social environmental factors appear to play a role.

Differential diagnosis. Other medical conditions; schizophrenia; anxiety disorder; panic disorder; depression; pain disorder; sexual dysfunction; dissociative disorder; hypochondriasis.

Classification criteria.

(a) Required for medical diagnosis: Recurring, multiple physical symptoms unexplained by a known medical condition or substance use, beginning before age 30, occurring over several years, resulting in treatment-seeking or significant impairment socially or occupationally. Additionally, the following findings must have occurred at some time since onset: four pain symptoms; two gastrointestinal symptoms; one sexual symptom; one pseudoneurological symptom (e.g., pseudoseizures).

(b) Required to attribute a voice problem to the medical diagnosis: Significant voice symptoms and usually signs in the context of other somatic complaints, consistent with Somatization Disorder and not wholly attributable to other causes.

Severity criteria:

(a) Medical: See Introduction

(b) Vocal: See Introduction

6012. Conversion Disorder (historically "hysteria" or Briquet's syndrome)

Essential features. The primary defining feature is non-trivial, significant deficit in voluntary motor or sensory function (e.g., pseudoparalysis, aphonia, pseudoblindness, pseudoseizures, tremor) not fully explained by a medical condition. Vegetative functions are typically intact.

Associated features. Symptoms or signs occur following stress or conflict, and are not attributable to malingering, substance use, or a culturally accepted behavior within the individual's environment. The behavior causes significant clinical distress or impaired life functioning. Symptoms and signs are not restricted to sexual dysfunction or pain. Individuals may display surprising lack of apparent concern, or "*la belle indifference.*" The left side of the body is more commonly affected than the right.

Vocal impairment. Findings can range from dysphonia to odynophonia, vocal fatigue, and total voice loss. Vegetative vocal tasks remain intact (coughing, laughing, etc.). Typically, conditions affecting voice are not accompanied by other manifestations of conversion.

Aerodynamic characteristics. Variable. Minimum and average phonatory airflows may be increased, if vocal fold contact is incomplete.

Acoustic characteristics. Variable. When voice is present, fundamental frequency is often increased, perturbation is increased, and signal-to-noise ratio is reduced. However, aphonia is a common finding.

Age at onset. Onset is usually late childhood to early adulthood. However, younger and older onsets have been reported.

Course. Onset is typically acute. However, symptoms may increase gradually. Especially isolated symptoms tend to remit quickly. For hospitalized cases, remittance usually occurs within 2 weeks. Symptom recurrence occurs in some patients (between 1/5 to ¼ of patients, within 1 year). Prognosis tends to be good for aphonia, limb paralysis, and blindness. Prognosis is poorer for tremors and seizures.

Complications. A primary complication is incorrect medical diagnosis, followed by inappropriate medical or surgical intervention. Secondary complications occur in social and occupational functioning.

Predisposing factors. Data indicate that 64% of patients with conversion disorder have organic brain disorder, in comparison to 5% of control subjects. Additionally, some evidence suggests a genetic link (see familial pattern below).

Prevalence. Reports range from 15–22 cases per 100,000, to as much as 300 cases per 100,000 in the population.

Sex ratio. More common in females. Sex ratio is estimated between 2:1 and 10:1.

Familial pattern. Limited data exist suggesting an increased risk in individuals with family members having the disorders. Risk is increased for monozygotic but not dizygotic twins.

Differential diagnosis. Amyotrophic Lateral Sclerosis; anxiety, Bell's palsy, depression, Huntington chorea, hyperparathyroidism, myasthenia gravis, Factitious Disorder, spasticity, dystonia, organically based tremor.

Classification criteria.

(a) Required for medical diagnosis: Wholesale disruption in voluntary motor or sensory function (e.g., pseudoparalysis, aphonia/dysphonia, pseudoblindness, pseudoseizures, tremor) not fully explained by a general medical condition; symptoms or signs follow stress or conflict, and are not attributable to malingering, substance use, or socially sanctioned behavior; the problem causes significant clinical distress or altered life functioning; symptoms and signs are not restricted to sexual dysfunction or pain.

(b) Required to attribute a voice problem to the medical diagnosis: Significant disruption or loss of voice, satisfying criteria for conversion disorder, not wholly attributable to other causes. Confidence in the diagnosis is increased by evidence of intact vegetative laryngeal functions, and by rapid resolution with behavioral intervention. However, it should be noted that intact cough is neither necessary nor sufficient to attribute a voice problem to a conversion condition.

Severity criteria:

(a) Medical: See Introduction

(b) Vocal: See Introduction

6013. Pain Disorder

Essential features. The primary presenting factor is pain in one or more locations, without clear relation to a general medical condition. Pain causes significant distress or reduction in function in social or occupational domains. The condition may be acute or chronic.

Associated features. Psychological factors appear to play a role in onset, exacerbation, or maintenance. Pain is not attributable to malingering, mood disorder, anxiety, or psychosis, and does not satisfy criteria for dyspareunia (pain with sexual intercourse). In voice, the predominant feature is odynophonia or, more generally, laryngeal pain.

Vocal impairment. Odynophonia and laryngeal pain are predominant features.

Aerodynamic characteristics: Variable; may be unaffected.

Acoustic characteristics: Variable; may be unaffected.

Age at onset. The condition is seen in children as well as adults. Thus, onset at any age is implied.

Course. Acute pain usually resolves after brief duration. With chronic pain, a positive prognostic factor for recovery appears to be maintenance of consistent work schedule or consistent participation in scheduled life activities, without acquiescence to pain as a determinant of lifestyle.

Complications. Extensive or aggressive medical treatment with confounding side-effects, and habituation. Reduction in participation in life activities.

Predisposing factors. Cultural factors may influence the expressed perception of pain. Evidence showing nonspecific inflammatory changes throughout the GI tract indicates a role of immunomodulation. Emotional factors can increase muscular tension and thus muscular pains and headaches. Psychosocial factors include family history of anxiety, depression, and other psychiatric conditions, chronic illness in a parent, psychological stressors, and secondary gain.

Prevalence. 10–30% of children and adolescents experience headache or abdominal pain without detectable medical cause, at least once weekly. Estimates indicate that 10–15% of adults have some form of occupational disability due to back pain alone, within a given year in the United States.

Sex ratio. Females experience some chronic pain conditions more often than males (e.g., headaches, musculoskeletal pain).

Familial pattern. Increased frequency of depression, alcohol dependence, and chronic pain in first-degree biological relatives.

Differential diagnosis. Anxiety disorder, child abuse or neglect, conversion disorder. With regard to the voice, laryngopharyngeal reflux and Muscle Tension/Adaptive Dysphonia (8020) must be ruled out.

Classification criteria.

(a) Required for medical diagnosis: The primary presenting factor is pain in one or more locations, without clear relation to a general medical condition. The condition may be acute or chronic; pain causes significant distress or reduction of function in social or occupational functioning; psychological factors appear to play a role in onset, exacerbation, or maintenance of symptoms; pain is not attributable to malingering, mood disorder, anxiety, or psychosis, and not does satisfy criteria for dyspareunia (pain with sexual intercourse).

(b) Required to attribute a voice problem to the medical diagnosis: The primary feature is odynophonia or laryngeal pain, independent of phonation and not attributable to other medical causes Laryngopharyngeal Reflux (2300).

Severity criteria.

(a) Medical: See Introduction

(b) Vocal: See Introduction

6014. Hypochondriasis

Essential features. Patient's significant preoccupation with, and fear of having one or more significant diseases, without medical basis, based on misinterpretation of bodily feedback. Preoccupation persists despite negative results of medical tests and reassurance. Beliefs around health status are not delusional, and cause significant distress or altered life functioning with duration of at least 6 months.

Associated features. Medical history is often related in great detail. Patients present a history of significant treatment-seeking behavior (peregrination), known commonly as "doctor shopping," with characteristic deteriorating relations with medical professionals, anger, and frustration. A history of multiple complaints, without medical basis, is common. Family life may become centered around the patient's problems. In voice, complaints may occur in the context of numerous other somatic symptoms, many or most without known medical basis.

Vocal impairment. Commonly, signs and symptoms point to the possibility of neurogenic disorder, without a clear, cohesive pattern consistent with known neurogenic conditions.

Aerodynamic characteristics: Variable.

Acoustic characteristics: Variable.

Age at onset. Information not available.

Course. The condition is usually intermittent.

Complications. Inappropriate, invasive treatments with side effects. Disrupted familial, social, and occupational function.

Predisposing factors. Neurochemical deficiencies and selected other somatoform disorders may co-occur, as for depression and anxiety. This finding may explain co-morbidity of the conditions as well as effectiveness of single treatments affecting the whole spectrum of conditions (e.g., selective serotonin reuptake inhibitors). Additionally, psychosocial factors appear to increase the risk of hypochondriasis, including negative parental attitude toward illness, and prior illness in the patient.

Prevalence. 3%–5% of cases in medical settings correspond to hypochondriasis. Rates are similar in the United States and internationally.

Sex ratio. Appears to occur equally in males and females.

Familial pattern. Unknown.

Differential diagnosis. Anxiety, conversion disorder, depression, personality disorder, schizophrenia.

Classification criteria.

(a) Required for medical diagnosis: Preoccupation with having serious medical disease, based on misinterpretation of somatic information; preoccupation persists despite negative results of medical tests and reassurance; beliefs around health status are not delusional; beliefs cause significant distress or altered life functioning; duration of at least 6 months; condition is not better as corresponding to Generalized Anxiety Disorder, Obsessive-Compulsive Disorder, Panic Disorder, Major Depression, Separation Anxiety, or other Somatoform Disorder.

(b) Required to attribute a voice problem to the medical diagnosis: Significant preoccupation with having serious disease affecting voice, in the absence of physical confirmation; general profile consistent with hypochondriasis.

Severity criteria.

(a) Medical: See Introduction

(b) Vocal: See Introduction

6020. Factitious Disorders

Essential features. Purposeful production or imitation of medical signs or symptoms. Munchausen's syndrome, which some authors consider a subtype of Factitious Disorders, is distinguished by particularly virulent involvement with the factitious condition, dangerous attempts to inflict injury or the appearance of disease, peregrination (traveling from doctor to doctor to seek treatment), even across cities and countries, and the presence of false claims about associations with famous individuals, personal credentials, and exceptional accomplishments.

Associated features. In Factitious Disorders, the patient's responses to in-depth questions about signs and symptoms may be vague and inconsistent. When the predominant feature of the complaints is psychological symptoms, the patients may respond to factual queries with approximate answers (the *Diagnostic and Statistical Manual of Mental Disorders-IV* gives the example that the response to a query about the product of 8 times 8 might be 65). Also, the patient may use a variety of substances to induce symptoms, such as psychoactive substances. When the condition predominantly focuses on physical signs and symptoms, substance abuse and inappropriate use of analgesics may be present.

Vocal impairment. Vocal impairments may be included as feigned symptoms and signs of disease.

Aerodynamic characteristics: Variable.

Acoustic characteristics: Variable.

Age at onset. Usually first occurs in early adult age, often following hospitalization for a medical or other mental disease.

Course. The condition is usually chronic.

Complications. Extensive inappropriate medical treatments; classic "gridiron abdomen" from multiple inappropriate surgeries. Numerous hospitalizations across the lifespan are not uncommon. Patients may change from doctor to doctor, and may change cities and even countries to continue their pattern of medical treatment-seeking.

Predisposing factors. Not well understood. Some speculation indicates history of neglect or abandonment as a risk factor. Other hypotheses about risk factors point to possible masochism, desire to be the center of attention, to be dependent, poor self-esteem and vulnerability, the need to feel superior to authority figures such as physicians by duping them; grudge against medical professionals or history of personal relations with medical professional; personality disorder (borderline, narcissistic, antisocial personality disorder in particular).

Frequency. Reliable estimates are not available. Specific sites (e.g., large teaching hospital in Canada) have indicated a frequency of 0.8% of cases involving Factitious Disorder. In a clinic in Australia, 1.5% of infants had Factitious Disorder by parental or other proxy.

Sex ratio. Appears more common in males than females.

Familial pattern. Unknown.

Differential diagnosis. Actual medical conditions or other psychiatric illness (Delusional Disorder, Depression, Schizophrenia); malingering, which has external (e.g., financial) incentive, whereas Factitious Disorder has internal incentive.

Classification criteria.

(a) Required for medical diagnosis: Purposeful production or imitation of physical or mental disease; motivation to assume the role of a sick person; lack of external motivation for the behaviors (financial gain, avoidance of responsibility, improvement in physical status, as with malingering). Additional criteria for Munchausen's syndrome include especially consuming preoccupation with the feigned illness and pursuit of medical treatment; significant attempts to actually generate dangerous medical conditions, peregrination, and grandiosity regarding accomplishments, relationships with famous individuals, credentials, etc.

(b) Required to attribute a voice problem to the medical diagnosis: Purposeful production of voice disturbance, satisfying criteria for Factitious Disorder in general. Normal voice under sodium amytal interview may be a useful adjunct to classification.

Severity criteria.

(a) Medical: See Introduction

(b) Vocal: See Introduction

6030. Selective Mutism (previously Elective Mutism)

Essential features. Withholding of oral communication (speech) in specific social settings, in the presence of normal laryngeal structure, and normal voice function in most settings.

Associated features. Psycho-social problems, social isolation, embarrassment, clinging, compulsivity, temper tantrums, defiant or oppositional actions, especially within the home environment.

Co-morbidities in children may include enuresis, encopresis, abnormal electroencephalography results, and possibly speech and language disorders.

Vocal impairment. Voice is characteristically normal when phonation is present.

Aerodynamic characteristics: Normal, when voice is present.

Acoustic characteristics: Normal, when voice is present.

Age of onset. Usually prior to age 5. However, the problem may not be addressed clinically until school age. May occur at other times during the school-age years in response to traumatic events. Can occur in adults.

Course. Sometimes the condition persists for only a few months. However, without intervention, it may persist for years.

Complications. Social isolation; teasing by peers; educational difficulties.

Predisposing factors. Stressful or humiliating experience in school or pre-school.

Frequency. The condition occurs in less than 1% of children presenting to mental health centers.

Sex ratio. Somewhat greater frequency in females.

Familial pattern. The condition is more common in families with first- and second-degree relatives who have panic or other anxiety disorders.

Differential diagnosis. Hearing loss; oppositional-defiant disorder; causes due to English as a second language and associated cultural factors; mental retardation; aphasia or apraxia; Mood Disorder; Somatization Disorder; Pervasive Developmental Disorder; Schizophrenia; other Psychotic Disorder; abnormal EEG; primary speech or language disorder that could account for the problem.

Classification criteria.

(a) Required for medical diagnosis: Reliable failure to speak in specified settings (e.g., school) in the context of speech occurring in other settings; the problem negatively influences educational, social, or occupational functioning; duration of 1 month or longer (excluding the first month in school).

(b) Required to attribute a voice problem to the medical diagnosis: Same as for medical diagnosis.

Severity criteria.

(a) Medical: See Introduction

(b) Vocal: See Introduction

6040. Anxiety

Anxiety encompasses a spectrum of conditions including Panic Attack, Agoraphobia (fear of open spaces), Panic Disorder Without Agoraphobia, Panic Disorder With Agoraphobia, Agoraphobia Without History of Panic Disorder, Specific Phobia, Social Phobia, Obsessive-Compulsive Disorder, Posttraumatic Stress Disorder, Acute Stress Disorder, Generalized Anxiety Disorder, Anxiety Disorder Due to a General Medical Condition, Substance-Induced Anxiety Disorder, and Anxiety Disorder Not Otherwise Specified. Of these, Posttraumatic Stress Disorder and Generalized Anxiety Disorder are probably those conditions most likely to have a causal relation to a voice problem. Accordingly, those conditions will be presented in this section.

6041. Posttraumatic Stress Disorder

Essential features. History of witness to serious events which threatened physical safety or life of self or others; the response was significant fear, helplessness, or horror.

Associated features. The original event is re-experienced chronically in one or more ways: recurrent intrusive memories of the event; recurrent dreams of the event which are distressing; sense of reliving the event; significant psychological distress in response to internal or external cues connected to the event; heightened physiological response to internal or external cues connected to the event; significant avoidance of stimuli connected to the event, or psychological numbing in response to those stimuli; persistent symptoms of heightened arousal not present prior to the event (e.g., sleep difficulties, irritability, attentional difficulties, hypervigilance, heightened startle response). Voice problems associated with Posttraumatic Stress Disorder may manifest as some form of Muscle Tension/Adaptive Dysphonia (8020), sometimes in extreme form up to and including aphonia.

Vocal impairment.

Aerodynamic characteristics: Variable.

Acoustic characteristics: Variable.

Age at onset. Any age, including childhood.

Course. Symptoms typically have onset within 3 months of the traumatic event. However, symptom onset may also occur with a delay of months or years.

Complications. Restrictions in educational, social, occupational, and familial functioning, which may be profoundly debilitating in some cases.

Predisposing factors. Witness of serious threat of physical harm to oneself or others, including threat or actual death.

Frequency. Lifetime prevalence of 8–10% of individuals in the general population. Studies of individuals who are at risk (e.g., veterans of combat, individuals exposed to volcanic eruptions, victims of violent crime) have indicated a prevalence ranging from 3%–58%.

Sex ratio. Females may have higher frequency of the disorder than males. Females are most likely to have the condition secondary to sexual assault; a more common source of the condition in males is exposure to combat.

Familial pattern. Unknown.

Differential diagnosis. Obsessive-Compulsive Disorder; Schizophrenia; malingering; substance-induced disorders; voice problems due to other causes.

Classification criteria.

(a) Required for medical diagnosis: History of witness to serious events which threatened physical safety or life of self or others; the response was significant fear, helplessness, or horror. The original event is re-experienced chronically in one or more ways: recurrent intrusive memories of the event; recurrent dreams of the event which are distressing; sense of reliving the event; significant psychological distress and/or heightened physiologic response to internal or external cues connected to the event; significant avoidance of stimuli connected to the event, or psychological numbing in response to those stimuli; persistent symptoms of heightened arousal not present prior to the event (e.g., sleep difficulties, irritability, attentional difficulties, hypervigilance, heightened startle response).

(b) Required to attribute a voice problem to the medical diagnosis: Voice symptoms and signs can be related to the medical condition, not wholly attributable to another condition.

Severity criteria.

(a) Medical: See Introduction

(b) Vocal: See Introduction

6042. Generalized Anxiety Disorder

Essential features. Extensive worry and anxiety fluctuating across numerous issues, on more than half of all days for at least 6 months. The individual has difficulty controlling the anxiety, which is accompanied by at least three of the following: restlessness, easy fatigability, difficulty paying attention, irritability, muscle tension, sleep abnormalities. Anxiety and worry are not limited to issues characteristic of other psychiatric diagnoses (e.g., fear of having a panic attack, social fear, fear of contamination, separation anxiety, fear of gaining weight, fear of serious illness, posttraumatic stress syndrome). The condition causes significant distress and negative influence in life functioning.

Associated features. The focus of the anxiety may shift across issues, but the general pattern of anxiety is persistent. Voice problems may occur as one manifestation of the disorder.

Vocal impairment. Data are not available for voice conditions specifically diagnosed as Generalized Anxiety Disorder. However, it is reasonable to assume that these voice problems may be mediated by muscle tension. Vocal impairment may involve dysphonia or aphonia, often without organic findings.

Aerodynamic characteristics: Variable.

Acoustic characteristics: Variable.

Age at onset. In the majority of cases, symptoms are reported to have initiated in childhood or adolescence (more often the latter). However, onset may also occur after age 20.

Course. Symptoms usually fluctuate across the lifespan. Symptoms tend to worsen during periods of stress.

Complications. Difficulty in social interactions and occupational functioning.

Predisposing factors. Although anxiety may have a familial pattern, no genetic basis has been found for Generalized Anxiety Disorder, specifically. Relative to voice, some reports indicate the possibility of a relation between state-trait anxiety, depression, and introversion plus neuroticism, and dysphonias without organic findings.

Frequency. 1-year rate is approximately 1–3%. Lifespan rate is about 5%.

Sex ratio. In children, frequency is about equal for males and females. However, in adolescence, females have greater frequency than males. For adults, about 55%–60% of individuals presenting clinically with the disorder are female. Epidemiological studies indicate an approximately two-thirds sex ratio in favor of females.

Familial pattern. Clear findings are not reported regarding a familial pattern in Generalized Anxiety Disorder.

Differential diagnosis. For medical diagnosis, the following conditions must be ruled out: Obsessive-Compulsive Disorder, Panic Disorder, Social Phobia, Attention Deficit/Hyperactivity Disorder; Posttraumatic Stress Syndrome; Bipolar Disorder; Depression; Dysthymia; Somatoform Disorder.

Classification criteria.

(a) Required for medical diagnosis: Medical diagnosis of the condition requires that the following criterion be met: extensive worry and anxiety fluctuating across numerous issues on more than half of all days for at least six months. The individual has difficulty controlling the anxiety, which is accompanied by at least three of the following: restlessness, easy fatigability, difficulty paying attention, irritability, muscle tension, sleep abnormalities. Anxiety and worry are not limited to issues characteristic of other psychiatric diagnoses (e.g., fear of having a panic attack, social fear, fear of contamination, separation anxiety, fear of gaining weight, fear of serious illness, posttraumatic stress syndrome). The condition causes significant distress and negative influence in life functioning.

(b) Required to attribute a voice problem to the medical diagnosis: Medical criteria must be satisfied for Generalized Anxiety Disorder, and voice problems not wholly attributable to other conditions.

Severity criteria.

(a) Medical: See Introduction

(b) Vocal: See Introduction

6050. Mood Disorders

This spectrum of psychiatric conditions includes Major Depressive Disorder, Dysthymic Disorder, Depressive Disorder Not Otherwise Specified, Bipolar I Disorder, Bipolar II Disorder, Cyclothymic Disorder, Bipolar Disorder Not Otherwise Specified, Mood Disorder Due to a General Medical Condition, Substance-Induced Mood Disorder, and Mood Disorder Not Otherwise Specified. Of these, probably the most common conditions to affect voice directly are Major Depressive Disorder (Recurrent) and Bipolar Disorders, which are discussed in the next sections.

6051. Major Depressive Disorder (Recurrent)

Essential features. History of two or more Major Depressive Episodes, separated by at least two months, involving five or more of the following, for most of the day during most days, during a 2-week period, including at least one symptom of depressed mood or anhedonia: reduced interest in pleasure in most or all activities; significant weight loss without dieting, significant weight gain, or change in appetite; insomnia or hypersomnia; increase or decrease in psychomotor function; fatigue or poor energy; feelings of having little self-worth or excessive guilt; poor concentration or indecisiveness; recurring thoughts of death, suicidal ideation, or suicide attempt. Symptoms cause significant disruption to life activities; symptoms are not attributable to effects of a substance or general medical condition; symptoms are not attributable to bereavement, and last for more than two months after the loss of a loved one.

Associated features. Voice problems can occur in conjunction with depression or their pharmacologic treatments. Also, secondary phonotraumatic lesions have been reported in some cases as the result of crying or sobbing.

Vocal impairment. Although specific data are not available, clinical observations suggest that voice problems having an etiological link to depression may be manifested by hypoadducted voice function, in conjunction with muscular hyper- or hypofunction depending on the characteristics of the depression.

Aerodynamic characteristics: Variable.

Acoustic characteristics: Fundamental frequency and intensity are reported to be decreased with depression.

Age at onset. Average onset occurs in the mid-twenties.

Course. Recurrence of depressive episodes may cluster during brief time periods, or years may intervene between recurrences. Among individuals who have a single depressive episode, about 50%–60% will have at least one additional occurrence.

Complications. Significant disruption often occurs in life activities, general health behaviors, and suicide. For voice, a complication may arise with the use of antidepressants, many of which are drying and thus may increase the risk of poor voice function and phonotrauma.

Predisposing factors. Genetic factors (see familial pattern below); disruption in serotonin (i.e., 5-HTP) in the central nervous system; disruption in norepinephrine and dopamine; learned helplessness.

Frequency. Approximately 10%–25% of women and 5%–12% of men have Major Depressive Disorder across the lifespan in the United States. Prevalence at a given point in time is 5%–9% for women, and 2%–3% for men.

Sex ratio. Sexes are equally affected in prepubertal children. In adolescence, females are affected at twice the rate of males. Risk across the lifespan is 10%–25% for women, and 5%–12% for men in the United States.

Familial pattern. The condition has 1.5–3 times greater likelihood in individuals with first-degree biological relatives with the condition. Risk increases for individuals who have first-degree, adult biological relatives with Alcohol Dependence, and children of individuals with Attention Deficit/Hyperactivity Disorder may have increased risk as well.

Differential diagnosis. Differentials for medical diagnosis of the condition include mood disorders due to central nervous system disease, such as Alzheimer's disease, neoplasm, inflammatory disease, sleep disorders (obstructive sleep apnea), infectious disease, pharmacologic etiology, endocrine disorders, substance use, abuse, or dependence, seasonal affective disorder, dysthymia, anxiety disorders, eating disorders, personality disorders, normal bereavement. The differential for attributing a voice problem to Major Depressive Disorder requires that the voice problem cannot be more parsimoniously attributable to another condition or disease.

Classification criteria.

(a) Required for medical diagnosis: History of two or more Major Depressive Episodes, separated by at least 2 months (five or more of the following, for most of the day during most days, during a 2-week period, including at least one symptom of depressed mood or anhedonia (inability to derive pleasure from normal day to day activities): reduced interest most or all activities; significant weight loss without dieting, significant weight gain, or change in appetite; insomnia or hypersomnia; increase or decrease in psychomotor function; fatigue or poor energy; feelings of having little self-worth or excessive guilt; poor concentration or indecisiveness; recurring thoughts of death, suicidal ideation, or suicide attempt. Symptoms cause significant disruption to life activities; symptoms are not attributable to effects of a substance or general medical condition.

(b) Required to attribute a voice problem to the medical diagnosis: Voice symptoms and signs must be attributable to one or more aspects of the disease, such as depressed physiological functioning related to anhedonia in communication, vocal tract drying due to antidepressant use, or phonotraumatic lesions secondary to crying or sobbing.

Severity criteria.

(a) Medical: See Introduction

(b) Vocal: See Introduction

6052. Bipolar I Disorder

Bipolar Disorders in general encompass a series of conditions including Bipolar I Disorder, Bipolar II Disorder, Cyclothymia, and Bipolar Disorder Not Otherwise Specified. Bipolar I Disorder itself, which is discussed in this section, encompasses six different sets of criteria, including Single Manic Episode, Most Recent Episode Hypomanic, Most Recent Episode Manic, Most Recent Episode Mixed, Most Recent Episode Depressed, and Most Recent Episode Unspecified. General information is provided about Bipolar I Disorder.

Essential features. Clinical course involves one or more Manic Episodes (period at least 1 week in duration involving unusually high, expansive, or irritable mood), and involving three or more of the following symptoms: exaggeratedly positive self-esteem or grandiosity, decreased sleep needs, pressed speech, flight of ideas, easy distractibility, exaggerated pursuit of goal-directed activities or physical agitation, increased involvement in activities of pleasure with potential for harm, or Mixed Episodes (period at least 1 week in duration involving criteria for Manic Episode and Major Depressive Episode, nearly daily. Moods alternate rapidly.)

Associated features. Disorganized thinking, disorganized behavior. Educational, occupational, social, and familial disruption. Other psychiatric conditions may co-occur, including Anorexia Nervosa, Bulimia Nervosa, Attention Deficit/Hyperactivity Disorder, Panic Disorder, Social Phobia, and Substance-Related Disorders. Voice problems may manifest as a sequelae of rapid, loud, and extended speech, culminating in phonotraumatic lesions. Risk of voice disruptions in general, and lesions in particular, is increased by the use of medications causing xerostomia (dry mouth), and physiologic excitability.

Vocal impairment. Hyperfunction and phonotraumatic lesions may be a sequelae of Bipolar Disorder. Additionally, the risk of voice disruptions and phonotrauma is increased with the use of drying medications causing xerostomia.

Aerodynamic characteristics: Variable.

Acoustic characteristics: Variable.

Age at onset. Childhood to age 50 years. Average age of onset is 21 years, with most cases commencing between age 15–19 years.

Course. The disorder is recurrent. Most manic episodes occur soon before or soon after a Major Depressive Episode. The number of manic and major depressive episodes across the lifespan is greater for Bipolar I Disorder than for Major Depressive Disorder. Suicide is an extreme consequence of the condition (see complications).

Complications. Significant disruption in occupational, social, familial, and life functioning. About 25%–50% of people with manic-depressive illness (Bipolar Disorder) attempt suicide; 11% achieve it.

Predisposing factors. Although specific biological markers have not been found, genetic studies consistently implicate a genetic component to the disease (see familial pattern).

Frequency. Occurrence of bipolar disorders in general, across the life-span, is 1%–1.6%.

Sex ratio. Equal distribution across the sexes. However, females are more likely to experience rapid cycling bipolar disorder (4 or more cycles annually), as compared to men.

Familial pattern. Individuals with first-degree relatives having the disease have a seven-fold increase of risk for the disease, in comparison to the remainder of the population.

Differential diagnosis. Differentials for the medical diagnosis include: Anxiety Disorders, Hyperthyroidism, Posttraumatic Stress Disorder, Systemic Lupus Erythematosus. The primary differential required to attribute a voice disorder to Bipolar disease is idiopathic (non-psychogenic) hyperfunction.

Classification criteria.

(a) Required for medical diagnosis: Clinical course involves one or more Manic Episodes (period at least one week in duration involving unusually high, expansive, or irritable mood, and involving three or more of the following symptoms: exaggeratedly positive self-esteem or grandiosity, decreased sleep needs, press of speech, flight of ideas, easy distractibility, exaggerated pursuit of goal-directed activities or physical agitation, increased involvement in activities of pleasure with potential for harm), or Mixed Episodes (period at least one week in duration involving criteria for Manic Episode and Major Depressive Episode, nearly daily. Moods alternate rapidly.)

(b) Required to attribute a voice problem to the medical diagnosis: The individual's vocal manifestations can be directly linked to Bipolar disease characteristics (e.g., loud, rapid, pressed speech for extended periods; pharmacologic drying).

Severity criteria.

(a) Medical: See Introduction

(b) Vocal: See Introduction

6060. Gender Identity Disorder

Essential features. An individual's desired vocal behavior is not congruent with the biological sexual characteristics present at birth. There is dissatisfaction with the voice and communication patterns that are biologically predictable and an attempt is made to assume the other gender role on a part-time or full-time basis. Transgendered individuals have a strong desire to live as a member of the opposite sex from their biologic orientation. Transvestite individuals may cross-dress for many reasons, but they do so for reasons that do not include feelings of gender dysphoria.

Associated features. Some individuals may retain their original genitalia and permanently or temporarily cross-dress. Other individuals may undergo sexual reassignment surgery and hormone treatments. Sexual orientation may or may not change. A small percentage of male-to-female transsexuals undergo vocal fold surgery. Virtually all female-to-male transsexuals experience virilization as a result of hormonal therapy.

Vocal Impairment.
Adult male to female: Biologic males who desire to appear female. The following characteristics represent initial status prior to attempts to modify voice.

> *Aerodynamic characteristics:* Average phonatory airflow is usually too low in comparison to the target female voice.

> *Acoustic characteristics:* Fundamental frequency is low in comparison to the target female voice. Formant characteristics as well as suprasegmental features typically remain characteristic of male speech.

Adult female to male: Biologic females who desire to appear male. The following characteristics represent initial status prior to attempts to modify voice.

> *Aerodynamic characteristics:* Average phonatory airflow is usually too high in comparison to the target male voice.

Acoustic characteristics: Fundamental frequency is high in comparison to the target male voice. Formant characteristics may remain characteristic of female speech. However, this feature is less of a problem in gender identification than for male-to-female transsexuals.

Age of onset. Initial signs may manifest in childhood, adolescence, or adulthood.

Course. Dysphoria, or dissatisfaction with the original gender role, is usually experienced for many years prior to a decision to make a semi-permanent or permanent change to the other gender. It is common practice for physicians to require a candidate for sexual reassignment surgery to live full-time in the other role for at least 1–2 years prior to surgery. Voice therapy may be required, even after surgery, to achieve appropriate vocal behaviors. Treatment typically includes psychological intervention, medical therapy, and possibly surgery.

Complications. Cognitive and linguistic differences, together with nonverbal differences, complicate the process of learning to communicate in a different gender role. Rejection by family, societal pressures, and employment problems are frequently encountered. Vocal fold surgery inconsistently results in the desired voice changes due to poor mood control.

Predisposing factors. Unknown.

Frequency. 3–5% of Americans cross-dress (transvestitism). A very small fraction of individuals undergo sexual reassignment surgery (gender dysphoria). According to some European studies, approximately 1 per 30,000 adult males and 1 per 100,000 adult females consider surgical sexual reassignment.

Sex ratio. Higher incidence in biologic males (see above).

Familial pattern. Unknown.

Differential diagnosis. Biologic condition suggesting unclear gender.

Classification criteria.

(a) Required for medical diagnosis: Patients who seek treatment are self-identified as having dysphonia associated with gender dysphoria.

(b) Required to attribute a voice problem to the medical diagnosis: Voice characteristics inconsistent with desired gender.

Severity criteria.

(a) Medical: See Introduction

(b) Vocal: See Introduction

6070. Psychogenic Polydipsia (Compulsive Polydipsia, Obsessive Polydipsia, Psychotic Polydipsia)

Essential features. Polydipsia is a condition involving excess intake of fluids, whereby intake exceeds the kidneys' excretion capacity. A consequence is hyponatremia or "water intoxication," which involves a decrease in serum sodium levels and can be fatal. Psychogenic polydipsia is associated with psychological or psychiatric causes. Patients with psychogenic polydipsia may be hypervolemic or euvolemic. Hypervolemic hyponatremia involves an increase in total body sodium, but greater increase in total body water. Extracellular fluids are increased, producing edema. Euvolemic hyponatremia involves an increase in total body water, with normal total sodium amounts.

Associated features. Consequences of hyponatremia in general may include apathy, agitation, lethargy, difficulty concentrating, anorexia, headache, nausea, confusion, fatigue, muscle cramps, seizures, coma, hyponatremic encephalopathy, and death. Voice changes may occur, possibly due to increases in extracellular fluid (edema) or neurological changes.

Vocal impairment. Vocal impairment may be seen by non-specific dysphonia, possibly due to vocal fold edema.

Aerodynamic characteristics. Unknown.

Acoustic characteristics. Unknown.

Age at onset. May occur at any age. The risk of hyponatremia in general is increased in infants, particularly when given tap water to treat gastroenteritis, and also elderly individuals, who have a decreased sense of thirst and may have medical conditions complicating polydipsia.

Course. Psychogenic polydipsia can lead to hyponatremia when free water intake occurs in excess of 10–15 liters of water daily, even if solute intake is normal. Hyponatremia more generally may be acute or chronic. Acute cases involve a decrease in sodium levels over a 24- to 48-hour period, possibly producing severe cerebral edema, brainstem herniation, and death. Chronic cases involve sodium decreases over days or weeks, in which case the brain generally compensates by extruding solutes and fluid to extracellular space. This mechanism reduces the diversion of free water into intracellular space, and symptoms are considerably milder compared to a similar level of acute hyponatremia.

Complications. Extreme complications include seizure and death.

Predisposing factors. Intake of 10–15 liters of free water daily, even with normal solute intake, is a risk factor for psychogenic polydipsia. Schizophrenia is the highest-risk psychiatric diagnosis for the condition. Other psychiatric risk factors include manic-depressive psychosis, psychosis with childhood onset, depression with psychosis, mental retardation, alcohol abuse, organic syndromes affecting mental processes, and personality disorders.

Frequency. Data indicate that psychogenic polydipsia occurs in more than 20% of inpatients in psychiatric facilities. Of those cases, approximately 5% appear to develop hyponatremia.

Sex Ratio. Unknown.

Familial pattern. Unknown.

Differential diagnosis. Polydipsia and hyponatremia from non-psychogenic causes (e.g., as associated with athletic activity).

Classification criteria.

(a) Required for medical diagnosis: Medical diagnosis of psychogenic polydipsia has traditionally lacked uniform criteria. However, a 17-item Polydipsia Screening Tool may be used that has been tested for reliability and validity (Reynolds, Schmid, & Broome, 2004). According to that tool:

> *High risk for psychogenic polydipsia* is seen with an increase in weight of at least 5% from morning to evening, and with morning urine specific gravity ≤ 1.008.

> *Moderate risk for psychogenic polydipsia* is seen with morning urine specific gravity ≤ 1.008, plus any of the following findings: tardive dyskinesia, smoking, consistently carrying around large cups with fluid, patient seen to be drinking from unconventional sources (e.g., faucet, toilet, shower head, fish tank), preferring fluids to food, frequent bathroom visits, socially unacceptable voiding (e.g., hallways), new onset nighttime incontinence, wearing extra clothing in the afternoon or sitting on radiator for warmth, afternoon behavior deterioration (irritability, anger, slurred speech, pacing, striking out, yelling, otherwise disruptive), distended abdomen, vomiting clear liquids, sweating, watery stools.

> *Low risk for psychogenic polydispia* is seen with three or more risk factors noted above, beyond evening weight gain and low morning specific urine concentrations.

> Medical diagnosis of hyponatremia requires serum sodium level < 135 mEq/L. Severe hyponatremia is seen with serum level < 120 mEq/L.

(b) Required to attribute a voice problem to the medical diagnosis: Dysphonia or other vocal disturbance varying with polydipsic behavior, not wholly attributable to other causes.

Severity criteria.

(a) Medical: see classification criteria for high, moderate, and low risk.

(b) Vocal: See Introduction

6080. Psychogenic Tremor-Like Voice Fluctuations

Essential features. This condition usually occurs in concert with other indicators of conversion disorder or multiple somatizations. This form of tremor is characterized by a sudden onset in one or more limbs without progression in severity. The tremor may spread to other body parts over a short duration in the absence of other neurological signs, and does not respond to pharmaceutical intervention. This form of tremor presents with a range of frequency rates within and across subjects and tasks. Tremor amplitudes tend to be large. They may be observed as both resting and postural/kinetic tremors atypical of any other form of tremor. Clinical observation and electrophysiologic testing in limbs typically describe a large-amplitude tremor associated with simultaneous activation of antagonistic muscles of the tremulous limb. Observations of this type are considered a necessary finding for clinical diagnosis in limbs. Diagnostic criteria for this form of tremor in voice are presently unclear. However, presence of psychogenic tremor in limbs, in conjunction with voice tremor, would increase confidence that the voice tremor is also psychogenic.

Associated features. The condition may reduce or disappear when the patient is not observed. The tremor in a resting limb will also decrease or entrain to the rate of finger tapping in the opposite limb. The amplitude and frequency of the tremor may demonstrate various patterns during electromyographic recordings. Adding weight or resistance to an affected limb results in increased amplitude of tremor atypical of organic tremors (e.g., decreased amplitude would indicate an organic tremor under these conditions). Individuals may slow their rate of speech to adapt to the perturbation of voice tremor during speaking. Similarly, individuals may prolong the duration of their vowels during speech. Individuals would be likely to report increased effort during speaking.

Vocal impairment. Vocal impairment is characterized by modulations of pitch, loudness, or both, during phonation at varying rates that may fluctuate under different conditions or at different times.

Aerodynamic characteristics: Unknown.

Acoustic characteristics: Frequency and amplitude variations should be observable from the acoustic trace, and may be variable across conditions and times.

Age at onset. Unknown.

Course. Sudden onset that may spontaneously resolve and then recur.

Complications. Impact due to impaired communication abilities can affect social, emotional, occupational, and physical well-being.

Predisposing factors. Conversion disorders and somatizations.

Frequency. Unknown.

Sex ratio. Unknown.

Familial pattern. Unknown.

Differential diagnosis. Abductor/adductor spasmodic dysphonia, dystonic tremor, Parkinsonian dysphonia, cerebellar disease, multiple sclerosis, laryngeal myoclonus, multiple system atrophy, enhanced physiologic tremor (8–13 Hz).

Classification criteria.

(a) Required for medical diagnosis: Modulation of pitch at varying rates across test conditions, or large-amplitude loudness modulations, during phonation. Presence of conversion disorder or history of somatizations, as well as co-occurring psychogenic limb tremor increase confidence in the diagnosis. Fiberoptic nasolaryngoscopy is useful to observe the degree of involvement in the larynx during both quiet breathing and during voice production and speaking. Distraction of the patient may result in decreased amplitude or disappearance of the tremor. Entrainment of voice tremor may be observed during finger tapping.

(b) Required to attribute a voice problem to the medical diagnosis: Same as for medical diagnosis.

Severity criteria.

(a) Medical: See Introduction

(b) Vocal: See Introduction

7000. NEUROLOGICAL DISORDERS AFFECTING VOICE

Many neurological disorders that affect voice may also affect speech. This relationship is applicable in more cases involving central nervous system disorders than it is to peripheral nervous system disorders. However, even with peripheral disorders, speech and voice may be affected, as with Myasthenia Gravis (7150). Whenever a neurologic condition is suspected, not only voice but also speech should be examined carefully.

7100. Peripheral Nervous System Pathology

7110. Superior Laryngeal Nerve (SLN) Pathology

Essential features. Absent or abnormal function of either the internal or external branches of the superior laryngeal nerve.

Internal branch. The essential feature of damage to the internal branch is sensory loss to the laryngeal vestibule and vocal folds as well as to the pharynx. Due to the innervation patterns, substantial sensory loss in the larynx or pharynx typically occurs when the internal branch is damaged bilaterally or if there is central involvement.

External branch. The essential feature of damage to the external branch is motor impairment of the inferior constrictor muscle and the cricothyroid muscle, which lengthens the vocal fold. Therefore, during attempts to produce high pitches, unilateral impairment of the external branch may be evidenced by rotation of the larynx off the midline. However, MRI imaging and other biomechanical data that describe the basis for this rotation are lacking, and signs of laryngeal rotation may be subtle and difficult to discriminate clinically.

Associated features.

Internal branch. The most common complaints are persistent cough, globus sensation, or a sense of irritation of the larynx and pharynx. In the event of bilateral sensory changes, laryngeal bolus penetration may occur without laryngeal response during deglutition. However, this condition is rare.

External branch. Associated findings may include reduced frequency and intensity ranges, and vocal fatigue. Also, there may be impairments in pharyngeal bolus transit, or reduced opening of the upper esophageal sphincter during swallowing.

Vocal impairment. The degree of vocal impairment may depend on the degree of impairment to one or both branches of the SLN.

Internal Branch: No predictable vocal impairment from unilateral damage to this branch.

External Branch: Reduced frequency and intensity ranges, vocal fatigue, and loss of pitch control, especially in higher ranges. Impairment may be more noticeable in professional voice users (e.g., singers).

Aerodynamic characteristics: Potentially increased airflow.

Acoustic characteristics: Reduced upper range(s) of fundamental frequency and intensity may occur.

Age at onset. SLN paresis or paralysis may occur at any age.

Course. Injury to the SLN may occur suddenly in the case of mechanical trauma (e.g., surgery) or progressively, in the case of disease processes (possibly viral, tumor, or an axonal neuropathy). The course of recovery following SLN paresis or paralysis is not known.

Complications. Silent aspiration or persistent cough only in the event of bilateral involvement of the superior laryngeal nerve or sensory loss of central origin. Aspiration with reaction can occur with unilateral involvement.

Predisposing factors. Surgeries to the head and neck; carotid, thyroid, cervical spine, and neck dissection; or other sources of mechanical trauma to the neck. Viral infection. Neuropathies, including hereditary motor and sensory neuropathy or Charcot Marie Tooth Type IIC.

Frequency. Unknown.

Sex ratio. Unknown.

Familial pattern. Motor and sensory neuropathies such as Type IIC have an autosomal dominant pattern of inheritance.

Differential diagnosis. Sensory afferent receptor disorder due to inflammation or tissue injury, vocal fold atrophy, scar, sulcus vocalis, recurrent laryngeal nerve paralysis or paresis, cricoarytenoid joint pathology, cricothyroid joint pathology, dysphagia due to other causes, Muscle Tension Dysphonia (8010), psychogenic dysphonia, and dysphonia due to other causes. In the event of bilateral sensory loss, consider a central disorder such as a brainstem stroke (e.g., Wallenberg).

Classification criteria.

(a) Required for medical diagnosis: Fiberoptic Endoscopic Evaluation of Swallowing Function with Sensory Testing may be performed to assess the internal (sensory) branch. Fiberoptic imaging of the larynx exhibiting a diagonal glottal line during phonation and asymmetry in vocal fold length and mucosal wave on stroboscopy will indicate external (motor) branch involvement. Laryngeal electromyography of the cricothyroid muscle can be used to verify the presence of electrical silence or evidence of other abnormal electrical muscle activity to assist in the diagnosis of external SLN paresis or paralysis (Sataloff, 2003). Complaints of globus, irritation, and persistent cough may indicate alteration in function of one side of the internal branch of the SLN, and thus increase confidence in the diagnosis.

(b) Required to attribute a voice problem to the medical diagnosis: Difficulties with pitch manipulations, especially in the higher pitch range, not wholly attributable to other causes, in conjunction with medical diagnosis of SNL paresis or paralysis.

Severity criteria.

(a) Medical: See Introduction

(b) Vocal: See Introduction

7120. Unilateral Recurrent Laryngeal Nerve (RLN) Paralysis

Essential features. Impaired function of recurrent laryngeal nerve (RLN) unilaterally, resulting in vocal fold immobility. For paralysis in the paramedian or lateralized position, incomplete vocal fold closure is likely during swallowing and phonation. If the superior laryngeal nerve is intact, the affected vocal fold may assume the paramedian position. If both the SLN and the ipsilateral RLN are impaired, the affected fold may assume a more lateralized position. For paralysis in the median position, dyspnea may occur with exertion or during voice use due to reduced airway opening.

Associated features. For paramedian or lateralized paralysis, breathy dysphonia, reduced loudness, reduced pitch and loudness ranges, loss of voice during shouting, complaints of vocal fatigue, and loss of air requiring frequent breaths during speech are expected. For paralysis in the median position, dyspnea may occur with exertion or during voice use due to reduced airway opening.

Vocal impairment. The degree of vocal impairment is related, in part, to the degree of lateral positioning and muscle atrophy of the immobile vocal fold. Patients often use large air volumes and abdominal pushing in attempt to increase vocal effectiveness, which may exacerbate the loss of air and augment the vocal impairment.

Aerodynamic characteristics: Average phonatory airflow is typically increased with paramedian and lateral paralysis. With median paralysis, airflow may be normal.

Acoustic characteristics: Average intensity is likely to be reduced with paramedian and lateral paralysis. Fundamental frequency may be increased or decreased. Fundamental frequency is often decreased shortly after onset of the condition, due to lack of muscle tone in the affected fold. However, some patients may use falsetto or high-pitched voice, possibly in an attempt to improve glottal insufficiency. Fundamental frequency is often increased in chronic cases, due to the conversion of muscle fibers to collagen (fibrosis), thus affecting the vibratory mucosa. Also, fundamental frequency in chronic cases may be increased due to passive stretching of the mucosa on the affected side.

Age at onset. RLN paralysis may occur at any age.

Course. Depending upon the etiology, may show recovery before 12 months. If paralysis remains after one year, it can be expected to persist.

Complications. Aspiration, Muscle Tension/Adaptive Dysphonia (8020).

Predisposing factors. Surgeries, trauma, or neoplasms of the head, neck, and chest (e.g., carotid, thyroid, esophageal, cervical spine, neck dissection, mediastinum, and cardiac). Other causes of RLN paralysis may include viral infection, congenital/genetic neuropathies, and idiopathic paralysis.

Frequency. Unknown. Among clinical cases, surgical trauma and malignancy of the head, neck, or chest are the most common causes of RLN paralysis. Other most frequent causes are viral infection, other neurological disorders, and idiopathic conditions. The left RLN is more commonly affected than the right, due to its longer course.

Sex ratio. Unknown.

Familial pattern. Most hereditary neuropathies have an autosomal dominant pattern of inheritance.

Differential diagnosis. Cricoarytenoid joint pathology (ankylosis or dislocation; see 3130) must be ruled out. Brainstem stroke (Wallenberg) can also result in unilateral vocal fold paralysis due to loss of motor neuron firing.

Classification criteria.

(a) Required for medical diagnosis: In cases of prolonged immobility and in the absence of other cricoarytenoid pathology, the diagnosis may be made visually using nasendoscopy and stroboscopy. Findings will show reduced or absent vocal fold abduction and adduction. Asymmetry of the mucosal wave can be seen on stroboscopy. Laryngeal electromyography can be used to verify the presence of electrical silence or evidence of other abnormal electrical muscle activity to assist in the diagnosis of RLN paralysis (Sataloff, 2003).

(b) Required to attribute a voice problem to the medical diagnosis: Weak, breathy, dysphonic voice associated with impaired adduction of one of the vocal folds that is not wholly attributable to other causes.

Severity criteria.

(a) Medical: The severity of laryngeal impairment is associated with the degree of lateral positioning and muscle atrophy of the immobile vocal fold in combination with compensatory strategies utilized by the patient. Severity of the global clinical picture can be described as:

Mild: Median: Vocal fold resides at midline.

Moderate: Paramedian: Vocal fold is slightly off the midline position (1–2 mm).

Severe: Lateral (cadaveric): Vocal fold is in an abducted position with resultant large glottal gap (3–4 mm).

(b) Vocal: See Introduction

7130. Unilateral or Bilateral Recurrent Laryngeal Nerve (RLN) Paresis

Essential features. Paresis refers to partial injury or neurological involvement of the axons in the recurrent laryngeal nerve. This condition can occur either unilaterally or bilaterally, and manifests as a reduction in movement or a reduction in vocal fold muscle tone or bulk. The essential clinical feature is a reduction in the amplitude or speed of adductory or abductory motion and/or a loss of bulk/tone of the vocal fold.

Associated features. Breathy dysphonia, intermittent pitch and voice loss, vocal fatigue, reduction in pitch and loudness ranges.

Vocal impairment. Vocal impairment depends upon both the degree and symmetry of vocal fold approximation, and the patient's compensatory adaptations. Some patients develop dysphonia in an attempt to overcome vocal fold weakness using increased supraglottic hyper-adduction on one or both sides. Expected findings for voice are re-duced pitch control, pitch breaks, reduced loudness, and breathy voice quality.

Aerodynamic characteristics: Average airflow and subglottic pres-sure are predicted to increase, depending on the degree and symme-try of vocal fold function.

Acoustic characteristics: Voice intensity and vocal intensity range may be decreased. Fundamental frequency may be increased, de-creased, or unaffected. Frequency range would be expected to de-crease. Acoustic findings will vary depending on the degree and symmetry of vocal fold approximation and the patient's compensa-tory adaptations.

Age at onset. Can occur at any age. However, weakness due to a gener-alized neuropathy is more likely to occur with aging past 60 years.

Course. Largely unknown. RLN paresis may completely or partially resolve within the first 12 months following onset.

Complications. Aspiration, Muscle Tension/Adaptive Dysphonia (8020).

Predisposing factors. Surgeries, trauma, or neoplasms of the head, neck, and chest (e.g., carotid, thyroid, esophageal, cervical spine, neck dissection, mediastinoscopy, and cardiac). Other causes of RLN paresis may include viral infection, hereditary neuropathies, or be id-iopathic.

Frequency. Unknown.

Sex Ratio. Unknown.

Familial pattern. Hereditary neuropathies have an autosomal domi-nant pattern of inheritance.

Differential diagnosis. Muscle Tension Dysphonia Primary; Muscle Tension/Adaptive Dysphonia Secondary (8010; 8020), scar, sulcus vocalis, vocal fold paralysis, central nervous system disease or event, cricoarytenoid joint ankylosis.

Classification criteria.

(a) Required for medical diagnosis: In cases of prolonged signs and symptoms, and in the absence of other cricoarytenoid pathology, the diagnosis may be made visually during nasendoscopy and stroboscopy. Findings will reveal asymmetries in abduction and adduction, and in vocal fold tension. Laryngeal electromyography can be used to verify the presence of electrical silence or evidence of other abnormal electrical muscle activity to assist in the diagnosis of RLN paresis (Sataloff, 2003).

(b) Required to attribute a voice problem to the medical diagnosis: Hoarse, weak voice consistent with physical findings and not wholly attributable to other causes.

Severity criteria.

(a) Medical: See Introduction

(b) Vocal: See Introduction

7140. Bilateral Recurrent Laryngeal Nerve Paralysis–Peripheral

Essential features. This condition is caused by bilateral vagal pathology affecting the RLN branch, or a peripheral neuropathy (axonal involvement) including hereditary motor and sensory neuropathy or Charcot Marie Tooth Type IIC. This condition manifests as bilateral immobility of the vocal folds.

Associated features. The nature and severity of associated features are dependent on the position of the immobile vocal folds affecting the size of the glottis. The most typical feature is inspiratory stridor when the vocal folds are paralyzed in the median position. In severe cases, airway obstruction may occur during bilateral vocal fold paralysis in that position. A breathy and rough voice quality, vocal fatigue, aphonia, and aspiration during swallowing may occur when the vocal folds are paralyzed in a lateral or paramedian position.

Vocal impairment. Vocal impairment is dependent on the position of the immobile vocal folds. The voice quality is breathy and rough, and pitch and loudness ranges are reduced when the vocal folds are para-lyzed in a lateral or paramedian position. In some instances, there may be aphonia. The voice quality is predicted to be minimally affected when the vocal folds are paralyzed in a median position.

Aerodynamic characteristics: Increased airflow may occur when the vocal folds are paralyzed in a lateral or paramedian position. Airflow and subglottal pressures may approximate normal when the vocal folds are paralyzed in a median position.

Acoustic characteristics: Though fundamental frequency may be normal, intensity range will be reduced.

Age at onset. This condition is more likely to occur in older age groups. For hereditary neuropathies, paralysis may be present from birth or childhood.

Course. A common scenario for bilateral vocal fold paralysis involves initial presentation of a weak, breathy voice quality, possibly with greater reduction in movement on the left side. As denervation persists, the vocal folds may come closer to the midline so that voice production is maintained, but the airway is severely compromised and stridor is consistent.

Complications. Airway obstruction or aspiration dependent on the position of the immobile vocal folds.

Predisposing factors. Surgeries or trauma to the head, neck, and chest (e.g., carotid, thyroid, esophageal, cervical spine, neck dissection, mediastinoscopy, and cardiac). Other causes of bilateral vocal fold pa-ralysis may include viral infection, brainstem compression (Arnold-Chiari Syndrome), peripheral neuropathies, and neoplasms.

Frequency. This condition is considered rare, with an estimated 1,500 cases per year in the U.S., most of which were due to trauma.

Sex ratio. No difference between males and females.

Familial pattern. Autosomal dominant pattern of inheritance in he-reditary motor and sensory neuropathy or Charcot Marie Tooth Type IIC.

Differential diagnosis. Psychogenic airway obstruction; paradoxical vocal fold motion; cricoarytenoid joint pathologies; with chronic development, may involve neurodegenerative diseases such as multiple systems atrophy, amyotrophic lateral sclerosis, or hereditary neuropathies.

Classification criteria.

(a) Required for medical diagnosis: Visualization of the larynx demonstrating impaired adduction and abduction of both vocal folds during inspiration and expiration, with no evidence of central nervous system involvement, nor cricoarytenoid joint pathology, and not wholly attributable to other causes.

(b) Required to attribute a voice problem to the medical diagnosis: Voice changes consistent with physical findings associated with bilateral vocal fold paralysis, not wholly attributable to other causes.

Severity criteria.

(a) Medical: See Introduction

(b) Vocal: See Introduction

7150. Myasthenia Gravis

Essential features. This condition is due to antibody binding to acetylcholine receptor sites at the neuromuscular junction of skeletal muscles resulting in rapid fatigue with movement and rapid temporary recovery. An alternative cause is genetic abnormality of the neuromuscular junction.

Associated features. This condition is most characterized by rapid fatigue of ocular, facial, bulbar, trunk, and limb muscles during movement with rapid temporary recovery upon cessation of movement. Extra-ocular muscles are most commonly affected by this condition. Rapid vocal fatigue within approximately five seconds of onset of phonation has been reportedly associated with this condition. In addition, swallowing difficulties and dysarthria have also been reported.

Vocal impairment. Vocal impairment from this condition is rare. When present, a breathy, weak voice quality with limited pitch and loudness variation may occur within approximately 5 seconds of onset of phonation.

> *Aerodynamic characteristics:* Airflow and subglottal pressure may decrease when the individual is symptomatic, due to global involvement of respiratory and laryngeal musculature.

> *Acoustic characteristics:* Fundamental frequency and intensity ranges may be reduced when the individual is symptomatic.

Age at onset. This condition can occur at any age; however, peak onset in females is in the 20s whereas peak onset in males is in the 50s and 60s.

Course. Extra-ocular muscle weakness is initially seen in 50% of cases and eventually occurs as a part of the profile in 90% of cases. Initial mild presentation increases in severity over weeks and months. A typical course involves spread of symptoms from ocular to facial and bulbar muscles and ultimately, muscles of the trunk and limbs. Concomitant disease or medications may trigger symptom crisis and acute respiratory failure. Patients generally improve with steroid treatment.

Complications. Respiratory failure. Current mortality rate is 3–4%.

Predisposing factors. The condition is thought to be idiopathic. However, infants having mothers with this condition may present with a transient syndrome.

Frequency. Two new cases per 1,000,000 annually.

Sex ratio. According to classic descriptions, this condition affects females more than males (3:2). However, with the current aging population, sex distribution is now equal.

Familial pattern. Infants having mothers with this condition may present with a transient syndrome.

Differential diagnosis. Amyotrophic lateral sclerosis, multiple sclerosis, psychogenic movement disorder, thyroid disease, Lambert-Eaton Myasthenic Syndrome.

Classification criteria.

(a) Required for medical diagnosis: A positive anti-acetylcholine receptor antibody test (positive in 74% of cases) and clinical improvement with a tensilon test.

(b) Required to attribute a voice problem to the medical diagnosis: Rapid decrements in vocal performance (speed, strength, rhythm) during the first few seconds following phonation onset, with temporary recovery in performance capabilities following brief rest.

Severity criteria.

(a) Medical: See Introduction

(b) Vocal: See Introduction

7160. Peripheral Neuropathy (Neuropathy, Charcot Marie Tooth IIC, or hereditary motor and sensory neuropathy)

Essential features: This condition is a familial demyelinating disease of motor and sensory nerves mostly affecting the longer nerves terminating in the leg and hand muscles, and the recurrent laryngeal nerve.

Associated features. This condition may be indicated by complaints of feet burning and fatigue. Laryngeal involvement may occur in either early or later stages of the condition. However, involvement of the hands and feet typically occurs in the early stages, whereas laryngeal involvement typically occurs in the later stages. Unilateral recurrent laryngeal nerve impairment may be evidenced by a breathy and weak voice quality. Bilateral involvement of the recurrent laryngeal nerve may result in inspiratory stridor related to impaired vocal fold abduction.

Vocal impairment. Vocal impairment is characterized by a breathy and weak voice quality with unilateral recurrent laryngeal nerve impairment. Minimal effect on voice quality is expected with bilateral recurrent laryngeal nerve impairment.

Aerodynamic characteristics: Increased airflow is predicted for unilateral recurrent laryngeal nerve impairment. Airflow may be unaffected, increased, or decreased with bilateral recurrent laryngeal nerve impairment.

Acoustic characteristics: Fundamental frequency may be increased, decreased, or unaffected with unilateral recurrent laryngeal nerve impairment, although intensity is expected to be reduced. Though fundamental frequency may be normal, intensity will be reduced with bilateral recurrent laryngeal nerve impairment.

Age at onset. Age 2–20 years for a juvenile form of the condition. Onset is typically between ages 20–40 for the adult form.

Course. Onset of this disease is associated with fatigue in the legs, difficulty opening jars with the hands, and maintaining a grasp. The left vocal fold is typically affected before the right vocal fold, due to the greater length of the left recurrent laryngeal nerve compared to the right. Bilateral involvement of the recurrent laryngeal nerve will produce stridor and breathing difficulties.

Complications. Respiratory obstruction.

Predisposing factors. May be hereditary in some but not all cases.

Frequency. Unknown.

Sex ratio. Equal across genders.

Familial pattern. Autosomal dominant.

Differential diagnosis. Amyotrophic lateral sclerosis, multiple sclerosis, multiple system atrophy, thyroid disease, Lambert-Eaton Myasthenic Syndrome.

Classification criteria.

(a) Required for medical diagnosis: Neurological examination and studies demonstrating denervation of nerves mostly affecting the longer nerves terminating in the leg and hand muscles, and the recurrent laryngeal nerve. Laryngeal examination reveals either unilateral or bilateral reduced vocal fold motion that is not wholly attributable to other causes.

(b) Required to attribute a voice problem to the medical diagnosis: Voice changes consistent with a reduction in vocal fold motion, not wholly attributable to other causes.

Severity criteria.

(a) Medical: See Introduction

(b) Vocal: See Introduction

7170. Enhanced Physiologic Tremor Affecting Voice

Essential features. This condition is an enhanced case of a normal physiologic tremor, present in the upper extremities. Normal tremor is described as a continuous oscillation of a limb or fingers. The tremor may be present at rest, posturally, or in action. Normal physiologic tremor can be enhanced by adrenaline upregulation (e.g., with increased anxiety), caffeine intake, or by thyroid hormones. Enhanced physiologic tremor is characterized as a static tremor of low amplitude and high frequency (8–13 Hz). Individuals usually report a history of less than 2 years since onset, no other history of neurological problems, and no familial history of a similar problem or disorder. When the condition affects the voice, a periodic modulation of pitch and loudness is expected at a rate between 8–13 Hz during sustained phonation of vowels.

Associated features. Electrophysiologic measures of this tremor will differ in frequency between sampled muscles from differing limbs or body parts. One contribution to the sampled frequency is the resonant frequency of the limb or body part (e.g., 25 Hz for the fingers, 6–8 Hz for the hand, 3–4 Hz for the elbow, and 0.5–2 Hz for the shoulder joint). The resonant frequency measured in a given limb or body part decreases when mass is added to the body part, or may increase with an increase in muscle stiffness. The physiologic tremor can be enhanced making it more visible or apparent, unrelated to a neurologic disease. This condition can be enhanced in several ways: adrenaline upregulation (e.g., with increased anxiety, as with stage fright), caffeine intake, thyroid hormones, medications (cold, asthma, sinus, antidepressant, or stimulant medications), withdrawal from alcohol or benzodiazepines, and medical conditions such as hypoglycemia and thyrotoxicosis. Correction of these conditions will result in resolution of the enhanced form of the tremor. Individuals with enhanced physiologic tremor affecting voice, report increased effort during speaking.

Vocal impairment. Vocal impairment is characterized by periodic modulations of pitch, loudness, or both during sustained phonation of vowels at a rate between 8–13 Hz.

Aerodynamic characteristics: Average airflow is predicted to be within normal limits.

Acoustic characteristics: Average fundamental frequency and intensity may range from normal to reduced during sustained phonation and connected speech.

Age at onset. Unknown.

Course. Onset may be sudden or progressive depending on the etiology. Correction of etiology typically leads to resolution of signs and symptoms.

Complications. Impact due to impaired communication abilities can affect social, emotional, occupational, and physical well-being.

Predisposing factors. Unknown.

Frequency. Unknown.

Sex ratio. Unknown.

Familial pattern. None.

Differential diagnosis. Abductor/adductor spasmodic dysphonia, benign essential tremor, psychogenic tremor, Parkinsonian dysphonia, cerebellar disease, multiple sclerosis, laryngeal myoclonus, multiple system atrophy, dystonic tremor.

Classification criteria.

(a) Required for medical diagnosis: Periodic modulation of pitch or loudness at a rate of 8–13 Hz during sustained phonation of vowels. Fiberoptic nasolaryngoscopy is useful to observe the degree of involvement during rest, speech, or vocalization as indicated by periodic movement of laryngeal, pharyngeal, palatal, or lingual structures associated with the perceived voice tremor.

(b) Required to attribute a voice problem to the medical diagnosis: Same as for medical diagnosis.

Severity criteria.

(a) Medical:

Mild: Regular modulations in voice loudness and pitch most evident during prolonged vowels and not detected in speech.

Moderate: Regular modulations in voice loudness and pitch that are mildly detectable during speech.

Severe: Regular modulations in voice loudness and pitch that are detected during speech and significantly alter the rate, prosody, and intelligibility of the individual's communication.

(b) Vocal: See Introduction

7200. Movement Disorders Affecting the Larynx

7210. Adductor Spasmodic Dysphonia (Spastic Dysphonia)

Essential features. The condition is a focal dystonia of the larynx, that is, an action- induced, task-specific movement abnormality characterized by intermittent hyperadduction of the vocal folds associated with perceived voice stoppages. This spasmodic hyperadduction of the vocal folds is most frequently associated with voiced speech sounds rather than voiceless speech sounds.

Associated features. This condition is characterized by strained, strangled, effortful phonation and intermittent voice stoppages, associated with overclosure of the vocal folds during production of vowels and glottal stops during connected speech. Dystonic vocal tremor or vocal tremor related to Essential Tremor (usually 6–8 Hz during sustained vowels) may co-occur in approximately 50% of individuals with this condition. See section 7240 for additional information on Essential Tremor also resulting in vocal tremor.

Vocal impairment. Vocal impairment is characterized as strained, strangled, effortful phonation and intermittent voice stoppages primarily on voiced speech sounds. In cases with severe hyperadduction of the vocal folds, voice loudness will be reduced. Symptoms typically improve with pitch elevation, singing, and during shouting. Vocalizations during laughter and crying are unaffected.

Aerodynamic characteristics: Average airflow varies within and across individuals; however, the literature reports an increased average glottal airflow in general, during sustained vowels and connected speech. More typically, these individuals exhibit large variations in airflow. Subglottal pressures would be predicted to show similar variations associated with intermittent overclosure of the vocal folds.

Acoustic characteristics: During connected speech, the following findings are typical: aperiodic segments defined as non-repetitive cycles, phonatory breaks greater than 50 ms, and frequency shifts of 50 Hz or more. Symptoms are less frequent on sustained vowels than in connected speech.

Age at onset. Onset most commonly occurs between ages 30–40. However, onset can be as early as 12 years or as late as 80 years.

Course. Symptoms frequently begin with a "catch" in the voice, and progress gradually over time. Infrequently, onset can be sudden. Initial voice symptoms may be reported to begin after an upper respiratory infection or related to a stressful life event or period. After onset, symptoms typically progress over a 1–2 year period and then plateau.

Complications. Highly negative sequelae commonly exist in social and occupational functioning due to the disease.

Predisposing factors. Other focal dystonias such as writer's cramp, torticollis, and blepharospasm may be present in affected persons or family members. Caucasians may have a greater probability of spasmodic dysphonia than Asian and Negro races.

Frequency. Estimated numbers of cases in the United States are 15,000, according to the National Spasmodic Dysphonia Association.

Sex ratio. 1.4:1, women-to-men.

Familial pattern. Rarely occurs in families, but in such cases transmission is from female to female.

Differential diagnosis. Muscle Tension Dysphonia Primary (8010), vocal tremor, mixed spasmodic dysphonia, abductor spasmodic dysphonia, irritable larynx syndrome, multiple sclerosis, cerebellar ataxia, and psychogenic dysphonia.

Classification criteria.

(a) Required for medical diagnosis: Adductory spasmodic voice stoppages associated with hyperadduction of the vocal folds during voiced segments of connected speech observed on fiberoptic nasolaryngoscopy. It is common for these individuals to produce a normal voice during sustained phonation of vowels, falsetto singing, and during vegetative laryngeal activities such as coughing and laughing. Non-response to behavioral intervention trials increases confidence in the diagnosis.

(b) Required to attribute a voice problem to the medical diagnosis: Perceived intermittent voice stoppages during voiced speech sounds in connected speech, consistent with visual evidence of hyperadduction of the vocal folds.

Severity criteria.

(a) Medical: See Introduction

(b) Vocal: See Introduction

7220. Abductor Spasmodic Dysphonia

Essential features. The condition is a focal dystonia of the larynx, that is, an action induced, task-specific movement abnormality characterized by intermittent breathy breaks during connected speech. These breaks are associated with prolonged voiceless speech sounds and intermittent involuntary abduction of the vocal folds is observable during fiberoptic nasendoscopy.

Associated features. Dystonic vocal tremor or vocal tremor related to Essential Tremor (usually 6–8 Hz during sustained vowels) may co-occur in approximately 50% of individuals with this condition. See section 7240 for more information on vocal tremor resulting from Essential Tremor. Often patients complain that speech is effortful or that they have difficulties with breathing control for speech.

Vocal impairment. Vocal impairment is characterized by intermittent breathy breaks typically associated with voiceless speech sounds. Patients may also exhibit upward pitch shifts prior to or following breathy breaks. Vocalizations during laughter and crying are unaffected.

Aerodynamic characteristics: Average airflow is predicted to be increased. More typically, individuals with this condition exhibit large variations in airflow across speech samples. Subglottal pressures would be predicted to show similar variations associated with intermittent abduction of the vocal folds.

Acoustic characteristics: During both connected speech and sustained phonation of the vowel /a/, the following findings are typical: aperiodic segments defined as non-repetitive cycles, phonatory breaks greater than 50 ms, and frequency shifts of 50 Hz or more, similar to findings for adductor spasmodic dysphonia. The breathy breaks are also associated with prolonged voice onset time following voiceless sounds during connected speech. In addition, loudness is predicted to be reduced due to breathy voice quality.

Age at onset. Onset usually between ages 30–40, but can begin as early as 12 years or as late as 80 years.

Course. Symptoms frequently begin with a "catch" in the voice and progress gradually over time. Infrequently, onset can be sudden. Initial voice symptoms may be reported to begin after an upper respiratory infection or related to a stressful life event or period. After onset, symptoms typically progress over a 1–2 year period and then plateau.

Complications. Impact due to impaired communication abilities can affect social, emotional, occupational, and physical well-being. Avoidance of the telephone is also frequently reported.

Predisposing factors. Other focal dystonias such as writer's cramp, torticollis, or blepharospasm may be present in the patient or members of the patient's family. Caucasians may have a greater probability of spasmodic dysphonia than Asian and Negro races.

Frequency. Unknown.

Sex ratio. 1.4:1, female-to-male.

Familial pattern. Rarely occurs in families, but in such cases transmission is from female to female.

Differential diagnosis. Muscle Tension Dysphonia (8010), vocal tremor, mixed spasmodic dysphonia, adductor spasmodic dysphonia, vocal fold bowing, vocal fold paresis, irritable larynx syndrome, and Parkinson's disease.

Classification criteria.

(a) Required for medical diagnosis: Intermittent breathy breaks associated with abduction of the vocal folds during voiceless consonants in connected speech observed during fiberoptic nasolaryngoscopy. Confidence in the diagnosis increases when voice is normal during all-voiced speech. It is common for individuals with this condition to produce a normal voice during sustained phonation of vowels, falsetto singing, and during vegetative laryngeal activities such as coughing and laughing. Non-response to behavioral intervention trials further increases confidence in the diagnosis.

(b) Required to attribute a voice problem to the medical diagnosis: Perceived intermittent breathy breaks following voiceless sounds in connected speech, consistent with visual evidence of intermittent vocal fold abduction.

Severity criteria.

(a) Medical: See Introduction

(b) Vocal: See Introduction

7230. Mixed Abductor/Adductor Spasmodic Dysphonia

Essential features. A rare form of spasmodic dysphonia characterized by a combination of intermittent involuntary abduction and hyperadduction of the vocal folds associated with breathy breaks and voice stoppages, respectively, as described for the abductor and adductor versions.

Associated features. Combined intermittent breathy voice breaks and voice stoppages associated with voiceless and voiced speech sounds, respectively. Individuals often complain of increased speaking effort and difficulties with breathing control for speech.

Vocal impairment. Vocal impairment is characterized by both intermittent breathy breaks and voice stoppages associated with voiceless and voiced speech sounds, respectively. Loudness may be reduced due to breathy voice quality during breathy breaks, and individuals may complain of increased effort during speech and difficulty with breathing control. Vocalizations during laughter and crying are unaffected.

Aerodynamic characteristics: Average airflow is predicted to be increased. More typically, an individual with this condition is likely to exhibit large variations in airflow during speech. Subglottal pressures would be predicted to show similar variations associated with intermittent abduction and overadduction of the vocal folds.

Acoustic characteristics: During both connected speech and sustained phonation of the vowel /a/, the following findings are typical: aperiodic segments defined as non-repetitive cycles, phonatory breaks greater than 50 ms, and frequency shifts of 50 Hz or more, as in adductor and abductor spasmodic dysphonia. The breathy breaks are also associated with a prolonged voice onset time following voiceless sounds during connected speech.

Age at onset. Onset usually occurs between ages 30–40. However, onset can occur as early as 12 years or as late as 80 years.

Course. Symptoms frequently begin with a "catch" in the voice and progress gradually over time. Infrequently, onset can be sudden. Initial voice symptoms may be reported to begin after an upper respiratory infection or related to a stressful life event or period. After onset, symptoms typically progress over a 1–2 year period and then plateau.

Some individuals believe that the mixed version of spasmodic dysphonia is due to compensatory behaviors that arise in response to primary adductory or abductory spasms. Thus, after a course of voice therapy, these individuals would exhibit adductor-type or abductor-type spasmodic dysphonia, rather than a true mix.

Complications. Impact due to impaired communication abilities can affect social, emotional, occupational, and physical well-being. Avoidance of the telephone is also frequently reported.

Predisposing factors. Caucasians may have a greater probability of spasmodic dysphonia than Asian and Negro races.

Frequency. Unknown, extremely rare.

Sex ratio. Unknown.

Familial pattern. Unknown.

Differential diagnosis. Muscle Tension Dysphonia (8010), essential tremor, abductor spasmodic dysphonia, adductor spasmodic dysphonia, vocal fold paresis, and irritable larynx syndrome. Must be distinguished from patients having adductor spasmodic dysphonia attempting to compensate by using a breathy voice, and from patients with abductor spasmodic dysphonia attempting to compensate by using glottal stops to initiate voicing.

Classification criteria.

(a) Required for medical diagnosis: Combination of adductory spasms associated with voiced speech sounds and abductory spasms associated with voiceless speech sounds during speech tasks, observed on fiberoptic nasolaryngoscopy. Normal voice in falsetto and during coughing, crying, and laughing may or may not be present. Non-response to behavioral intervention trials increases the confidence in the diagnosis.

(b) Required to attribute a voice problem to the medical diagnosis: Perceived intermittent breathy breaks following voiceless speech sounds and intermittent voice breaks associated with voiced sounds during connected speech, consistent with visual evidence of vocal fold abduction and adduction, respectively.

Severity criteria.

(a) Medical: See Introduction

(b) Vocal: See Introduction

7240. Dystonic Tremor Affecting Voice

Essential features. This condition is characterized as a postural/kinetic tremor and is typically observed in a body part affected by dystonia, although it can occur in isolation. When it affects the voice, this condition is manifested in the larynx, but can also involve pharyngeal musculature. Tremor is observed only during purposeful, or volitional activity such as sustained vowel production or speech, and is absent during quiet breathing. This tremor is described as exhibiting irregular amplitudes within speech tasks, and varied frequency below 7 Hz, across individuals. Voice tremor is best identified during sustained phonation of vowels.

Associated features. This condition is frequently associated with spasmodic dysphonia or other dystonias. Individuals may slow their rate of speech to adapt to the perturbation of voice tremor during speaking. Similarly, individuals may prolong the duration of their vowels during speech. Individuals report increased effort and decreased loudness during speaking. Individuals may also use compensatory postures to reduce the tremor amplitude.

Vocal impairment. Vocal impairment is characterized by periodic modulations of pitch, loudness, or both during sustained phonation of vowels at a frequency rate below 7 Hz. This condition is frequently associated with laryngeal dystonia, such as spasmodic dysphonia.

Aerodynamic characteristics: Average airflow is predicted to be within normal limits.

Acoustic characteristics: Average fundamental frequency and intensity may range from normal to reduced during sustained phonation and connected speech. Frequency and amplitude modulations may be captured in the acoustic signal.

Age at onset. Unknown.

Course. Similar to dystonia in that after onset, symptoms typically progress over a 1–2 year period and then plateau.

Complications. Impact due to impaired communication abilities can affect social, emotional, occupational, and physical well-being. Avoidance of the telephone is also frequently reported.

Predisposing factors. Caucasians may have a greater probability of laryngeal dystonia than Asian and Negro races.

Frequency. Unknown for laryngeal manifestation.

Sex ratio. Unknown.

Familial pattern. Unknown.

Differential diagnosis. Abductor/adductor spasmodic dysphonia, psychogenic tremor, Parkinsonian dysphonia, cerebellar disease, multiple sclerosis, laryngeal myoclonus, multiple system atrophy, enhanced Physiologic Tremor (8–13 Hz).

Classification criteria.

(a) Required for medical diagnosis: Periodic modulation of pitch or loudness at a rate less than 7 Hz during sustained phonation of vowels. Fiberoptic nasolaryngoscopy is useful to observe the degree of involvement in the larynx with onset of speaking or voice production, and the absence of involvement during rest breathing. Periodic movement of laryngeal structures, but not other vocal tract structures, in association with the perceived voice tremor.

(b) Required to attribute a voice problem to the medical diagnosis: Same as for medical diagnosis.

Severity criteria.

(a) Medical:

> *Mild:* Regular modulations in voice loudness and pitch most evident during prolonged vowels and not detected in speech.

Moderate: Regular modulations in voice loudness and pitch that are mildly detectable during speech.

Severe: Regular modulations in voice loudness and pitch that are detected during speech and significantly alter the rate, prosody, and intelligibility of the individual's communication.

(b) Vocal: See Introduction

7250. Essential Tremor Affecting Voice (Familial Tremor, Hereditary Tremor, Benign Essential Tremor)

Essential features. Essential tremor is a postural/kinetic tremor that typically begins in the hands and spreads to the legs, head, and speech mechanism. At onset, the tremor may be high frequency (8–12 Hz), but the frequency reduces to the classically described rate of 4–8 Hz in advanced stages. Tremor may be present during rest, particularly in cases involving head tremor. Voice tremor is identified during sustained phonation of vowels. Because voice is commonly affected later in the progression of this disease, tremor rates for voice are usually within the classic 4–8 Hz range. Pitch or loudness modulations may be involved, and may be secondary to contraction of muscles associated with the respiratory system (e.g., diaphragm, external intercostals, abdominal muscles), larynx, pharynx, soft palate, tongue, or jaw.

Associated features. Individuals may slow their rate of speech to adapt to the perturbation of voice tremor during speaking. Similarly, individuals may prolong the duration of their vowels during speech. Individuals report increased effort and decreased loudness during speaking.

Essential voice tremor may be somewhat reduced with alcohol and with beta blockers such as propanolol and primidone. However, it is more typical that pharmaceutical intervention does not affect the voice to the same degree as limbs and head tremors. Limb and voice tremors worsen with stress and fatigue. A head tremor may reduce when the head is supported, or the neck muscles are less active as when lying down or resting against a head rest.

Vocal impairment. Vocal impairment is characterized by periodic modulations of pitch, loudness, or both during sustained phonation of vowels, at a rate of 4–8 Hz. When severe, essential voice tremor can affect production of speech sounds and significantly reduce speech intelligibility.

Aerodynamic characteristics: Average airflow is predicted to be within normal limits.

Acoustic characteristics: Average fundamental frequency and intensity may range from normal to reduced during sustained phonation and connected speech. The specific tremor rate may vary with pitch and loudness. Tremor amplitude usually reduces at high pitches.

Age at onset. Onset is usually earlier in familial cases, beginning between ages 20–30 years, with a history of a mother or grandmother also having a shaky voice. Non-familial (sporadic) cases usually have a later onset, often in the 7th decade.

Course. Essential Tremor typically begins with a tremor in the hand(s) that may progress to the leg(s), head, and voice. Essential Tremor may gradually increase in severity with aging.

Complications. Impact due to impaired communication abilities can affect social, emotional, occupational, and physical well-being. Avoidance of the telephone is also frequently reported.

Predisposing factors. Essential Tremor is familial in 50–70% of cases.

Frequency. 415 per 100,000 people in the United States (for Essential Tremor in general). Unknown for laryngeal manifestation. 2–3 million individuals in the United States are diagnosed with Essential Tremor.

Sex ratio. High female predominance.

Familial pattern. See predisposing factors.

Differential diagnosis. Abductor/adductor spasmodic dysphonia, dystonic tremor, psychogenic tremor, Parkinsonian dysphonia, cerebellar disease, multiple sclerosis, laryngeal myoclonus, multiple system atrophy, enhanced physiologic tremor (8–13 Hz).

Classification criteria.

(a) Required for medical diagnosis: Periodic modulation of pitch or loudness at a rate of 4–8 Hz during sustained phonation of vowels, in conjunction with similar tremor findings in the hand(s), leg(s), or head. Fiberoptic nasolaryngoscopy is useful to observe the degree of involvement in the larynx, velum, and pharynx as indicated by periodic movement of these structures associated with the perceived voice tremor.

(b) Required to attribute a voice problem to the medical diagnosis: Same as for medical diagnosis.

Severity criteria.

(a) Medical:

> *Mild:* Regular modulations in voice loudness and pitch most evident during prolonged vowels and not detected in speech.

> *Moderate:* Regular modulations in voice loudness and pitch that are mildly detectable during speech.

> *Severe:* Regular modulations in voice loudness and pitch that are detected during speech and significantly alter the rate, prosody, and intelligibility of the individual's communication.

(b) Vocal: See Introduction

7260. Meige's Syndrome (Orofacial dystonia)

Essential features: This is a regional dystonia of the head and neck most commonly affecting the oral cavity, muscles of mastication, and eyelid muscles. Individuals with this condition are likely to exhibit increased blinking (blepharospasm) and involuntary jaw or facial movements (oro-mandibular dystonia). Movements may occur at rest or be movement induced, and may be task-specific. For example, movements only occur during speech and not during chewing. Symptoms are absent during sleep.

Associated features. Severe cases of dystonic muscle behavior may yield involuntary closing or opening gestures of the mouth, lip pursing, or tongue protrusion or retraction during speech. Muscle pain from cramping, and tooth injury from extreme jaw closing, frequently occur with this condition. Temporomandibular joint dislocation is common in jaw-opening dystonia. Pharyngeal dystonia may be present and, when severe, can obstruct the airway above the larynx constricting the posterior pharyngeal wall against the epiglottis. Dysarthria and dysphagia due to dystonic activity of the tongue or jaw muscles may occur. Additional associated focal dystonias are spasmodic dysphonia and torticollis. Sensory tricks applied to the affected structures such as touching the lips, chewing gum, touching the eyelid, or touching the chin may reduce dystonic muscle contractions.

Vocal impairment. The primary communication impairment is dysarthria. The vocal impairment, when present, is similar to impairment with adductor spasmodic dysphonia.

Aerodynamic characteristics: Unknown.

Acoustic characteristics: Unknown.

Age at onset. Typically middle-aged.

Course. Gradual onset with slow progression and then a plateau, similar to other dystonias.

Complications. Compromise in communication, aspiration, or airway obstruction.

Predisposing factors. Unknown. Genetic linkage under investigation. Many patients report symptoms starting after extensive dental work, ill-fitting dentures, or with speech overuse as with auctioneering or radio announcing.

Frequency. Unknown.

Sex ratio. Equal; may be higher in females.

Familial pattern. Unknown.

Differential diagnosis. Cortical spasticity, tardive dyskinesia, psychogenic dystonia.

Classification criteria.

(a) Required for medical diagnosis: Dystonic activity of the eyelid and oro-mandibular muscles. Movements are not modified by distraction or suggestion, and abnormalities are greater during purposeful movement.

(b) Required to attribute a voice problem to the medical diagnosis: Articulation deficits and/or cul-de-sac resonance, not attributable to other causes.

Severity criteria.

(a) Medical: See Introduction

(b) Vocal: See Introduction

7270. Tardive Stereotypies (Tardive Dyskinesia)

Essential features. This condition is characterized by involuntary movements affecting the face, tongue, lips, jaw, trunk, extremities, or larynx in patients treated with long-term neuroleptic medications.

Associated features. Dysphagia, dysarthria, motor speech disruptions, dysphonia, and intermittent involuntary vocalizations or stridor at rest. More globally, associated features typically include bradykinesia (abnormal slowness/rigidity) and hyperkinesia (purposeless movements). Movements are often more exaggerated at rest and reduced during speech.

Vocal impairment. May exhibit involuntary intermittent changes in resonance, voice pitch and loudness, and limited ability to perform rapid changes in voicing during speech.

Aerodynamic characteristics: Unknown.

Acoustic characteristics: Unknown.

Age at onset. Any age; Increased incidence with increased age and after prolonged use of phenothiazines.

Course. May be acute and resolve with withdrawal from medication, or may remain chronic.

Complications. Aspiration or weight loss from medication.

Predisposing factors. Mental illness requiring chronic administration of phenothiazines or D2 blockers. White elderly females appear to be more susceptible.

Frequency. 15–30% of all patients receiving long-term neuroleptic treatment develop tardive stereotypies.

Sex ratio. May affect women more frequently than men.

Familial pattern. None.

Differential diagnosis. Oro-mandibular dystonia, Meige syndrome, Huntington's Chorea, Tourette's syndrome, and Essential Tremor.

Classification criteria.

(a) Required for medical diagnosis: Uncontrolled oro-facial-mandibular movements secondary to neuroleptic treatment.

(b) Required to attribute a voice problem to the medical diagnosis: Uncontrolled hyperkinetic vocalization associated with phenothiazine treatment or D2 dopamine receptor blockers.

Severity criteria.

(a) Medical: See Introduction

(b) Vocal:

Mild: Involuntary voicing or some other involuntary motion at rest that does not interfere with speech or swallowing.

Moderate: Involuntary grunts or hums, movement of the face, lips, or tongue that draw attention and have some interference with speech and swallowing.

Severe: Speech unintelligibility and dysphagia because of interference of involuntary movements.

7280. Tourette's Syndrome

Essential features. Neurologic disorder characterized by involuntary motor and vocal tics with onset prior to 18 years of age, with most common onset occurring between 5–12 years of age.

Associated features. Frequently associated with complex generalized motor tics and ballistic movements. The tics may be temporarily suppressed, but the urge to tic continues. Tics are intermittent and more frequent when the individual is distracted. Tics may be reduced during speech. Complex vocal tics may include either repetitive involuntary productions or combinations of yells, grunts, shouting, barks, squeals, coughs, or squeaks as routinized sequences of non-speech productions (e.g., snorts, clicks, inspirations, glottal stops). Vocal tics can also include involuntary production of speech syllables, words, short phrases (including obscenities), or tunes. These types of tics are less frequent during conversational speech because they are suppressed during speech and occur at phrase boundaries. Cursing tics are relatively uncommon. There may also be compulsive ritualistic behaviors around certain activities.

Vocal impairment. The vocal impairment is characterized mostly by involuntary vocalization. If tics are loud barks or shouting, voice changes may occur secondary to vocal fold trauma.

Aerodynamic characteristics: Unknown.

Acoustic characteristics: Unknown.

Age at onset. Onset prior to 18 years of age, with most typical onset between 5–12 years.

Course. Progresses for the first 2 years and then remains chronic. Can reduce in adulthood.

Complications. Social maladjustment, depression, rage attacks, vocal fold phonotrauma, self-injurious behavior.

Predisposing factors. Family history of Tourette's syndrome or simple tics.

Frequency. Estimated at 1 in 1,000 children. Symptoms may disappear for some individuals in adulthood.

Sex ratio. More frequent in males (5:1).

Familial pattern. Thought to be an autosomal recessive genetic disorder with less penetrance in females than males.

Differential diagnosis. Must be differentiated from simple tics (although these may be an early sign of Tourette's syndrome), tardive dyskinesia, stuttering, chorea, cocaine seizures, and restless leg syndrome.

Classification criteria.

(a) Required for medical diagnosis: Repetitive motor and vocal tics for longer than one year with onset prior to the age of 18 years.

(b) Required to attribute a voice problem to the medical diagnosis: Same as for medical diagnosis.

Severity criteria.

(a) Medical:

Mild: a few intermittent vocal sounds that can be controlled for intervals.

Moderate: words or sounds that draw attention.

Severe: Frequent phrases and/or coprolalia (involuntary use of obscene words) that cannot be controlled.

(b) Vocal: Same as for medical.

7300. Central Nervous System Disorders

Hundreds of distinct, specific Central Nervous System (CNS) disturbances can affect the voice and other aspects of speech. Just a few examples of categories that could be added to the list here include corticobasal degeneration, Friedreich's ataxia, stroke syndromes, a number of unusual vascular disturbances (e.g., Mitochondrial Myopathy, Encephalopathy, Lactacidosis, Stroke, otherwise known as MELAS), tumor, trauma (e.g., Traumatic Brain Injury, surgical trauma), paraneoplastic cerebellar degeneration, multifocal leukoencephalopathy, meningitis, encephalitis, and hypoxic encephalopathy. Therefore, the list as currently given, is grossly incomplete. However, it would be unwieldy to try to list all CNS disturbances that might affect the voice and other aspects of speech.

In the presence of this quandary, we have elected to include conditions based on clinical prevalence in typical voice practices. However, the frequency of the conditions in the general population may be relatively small. In addition to excluding the aforementioned conditions and many others, the classification system does not include voice problems due to aphasia, apraxia of speech, or mutism associated with neurocognitive, language, or motor speech programming impairments.

7305. Amyotrophic Lateral Sclerosis (ALS; Lou Gehrig's Disease)

Essential features. This condition is characterized by upper and lower motor neuron involvement in the brain, brainstem, or spinal cord.

Associated features. Associated features include weakness of bulbar muscles, or of single or multiple limb muscle groups due to motor neuron death in the brainstem or spinal cord, respectively. Presentation is not always bilateral or symmetrical. Limb or tongue fasciculations are commonly seen. Distal limb weakness, or weakness and atrophy of the intrinsic hand muscles may also occur. Dysphagia and respiratory fatigue and failure occur in the terminal stages of the disease.

Vocal impairment. The bulbar form of this disease results in a breathy, weak, hypernasal voice with reduced average pitch and loudness and reduced pitch and loudness ranges. Slurred speech can also appear early in the disease. In such cases, voice changes, reduced vocal fold movements, and dysphagia may occur early in the disease. A tracheotomy may be required to provide an airway and enteric feeding may be required in later stages of the disease.

Aerodynamic characteristics: Unknown.

Acoustic characteristics: Voice frequency may be higher than normal in males. Fluctuations in frequency and intensity may be characteristic in patients within and across days, weeks, or longer intervals.

Age at onset. Between the 4th and 7th decades of life.

Course. ALS typically leads to death within five years. Fifty percent of individuals with ALS die within 18 months, 20% survive 5 years, and 10% live longer than 10 years after diagnosis. The bulbar form of ALS is the fastest progressing of the two types.

Complications. Dysphagia, aspiration pneumonia, respiratory insufficiency, inability to perform activities of daily living, and death.

Predisposing factors. Ten percent of ALS is familial; the disease is transmitted in an autosomal dominant fashion.

Frequency. 5 per 100,000.

Sex ratio. More males are affected than females (1.5:1).

Familial pattern. See Predisposing factors.

Differential diagnosis. Myasthenia Gravis, spinal-muscular atrophy, dementia in motor neuron disease, sarcoidosis (neuropathy).

Classification criteria.

(a) Required for medical diagnosis: The El Escorial World Federation of Neurology Criteria (1994) is used in diagnosis of ALS. Directly citing from this schematic:

"The diagnosis of ALS requires the presence of each of the following:
Lower motor neuron signs in at least two limbs
Upper motor neuron signs in at least one region (bulbar, cervical, or lumbosacral)
Progression of the disease defined as increasing symptomatic impairment by history. This may involve the same or new regions.
The diagnosis of ALS requires the absence of each of the following:

Sensory signs (except those attributable to aging)

Neurogenic sphincter abnormalities

Clinically evident peripheral nervous system disease with natural history of progress (e.g., diabetic polyneuropathy, hereditary polyneuropathy)

ALS-like syndromes:

Structural spinal cord lesions including spondylotic myelopathy

Multifocal motor neuropathy

Hyperthyroidism

Monoclonal gammopathy with an associated hematologic malignancy (e.g., lymphoma, myeloma [monoclonal gammopathy alone permitted])

Lead poisoning

History of radiation to the brain or spinal cord

Hexosaminidase A deficiency (patients under age 30)."

Wilbourn, A. J. (1994). Clinical neurophysiology in the diagnosis of amyotrophic lateral sclerosis: the Lambert and the El Escorial criteria. *Journal of Neurological Sciences.* 124 Suppl: 96—107. Reprinted with permission from Elsevier.

(b) Required to attribute a voice problem to the medical diagnosis: Flaccid or spastic dysarthria affecting voice. Findings may include "imprecise consonants, hypernasality, harshness, slow speech rate, monopitch, short phrases, distorted vowels, low pitch." (Darley, Aronson, & Brown, 1969).

Severity criteria.

(a) Medical: See Introduction

(b) Vocal: See Introduction

7310. Wallenberg Syndrome (Lateral Medullary Syndrome/Infarct)

Essential features. Lateral medulla infarct resulting in a unilateral vocal fold paralysis accompanied by Horner's syndrome, and contralateral numbness of the upper extremity due to vertebral artery occlusion or injury affecting the dorsolateral medulla oblongata.

Associated features. Associated features typically include vertigo, diplopia, ipsilateral facial pain and anesthesias, and dysarthria. Contralateral pain and thermal impairment over entire body and possibly the face may also be present. Dysphagia is typically due to neuronal loss in the medullary swallowing center and to hypopharyngeal sensory loss affecting swallowing. Ipsilateral ataxia may occur if the posterior inferior cerebellar artery territory is involved. Facial and palatal weakness may also be identified depending upon the extent of the lesion. Orthostatic hypotension is a frequent accompanying disorder.

Vocal impairment. The degree of vocal impairment is related, in part, to the degree of lateral positioning and muscle atrophy of the immobile vocal fold. Patients often use large air volumes and abdominal pushing in attempts increase vocal effectiveness, which may exacerbate the loss of air and augment the vocal impairment.

Aerodynamic characteristics: Average phonatory airflow may be increased with paramedian and lateral paralysis without adequate compensation by the mobile fold. With median paralysis, airflow may be normal.

Acoustic characteristics: Average intensity is likely to be reduced with paramedian and lateral paralysis. Fundamental frequency may be increased or decreased. Fundamental frequency is often decreased shortly after onset of the condition, due to lack of muscle tone in the affected fold. Fundamental frequency is often increased in chronic cases.

Age at onset. Typically in the 6th and 7th decades.

Course. May show some initial spontaneous recovery, often with residual neurologic deficits.

Complications. Aspiration pneumonia due to dysphagia.

Predisposing factors. Transient ischemic attacks, arteriosclerosis, hypertension.

Frequency. Rare.

Sex ratio. More frequent in males.

Familial pattern. None.

Differential diagnosis. Benign positional vertigo, vertebral artery dissection, labyrinthitis, multiple sclerosis, stroke, vestibular disease, idiopathic vocal fold paralysis, peripheral recurrent nerve injury.

Classification criteria.

(a) Required for medical diagnosis: Although Magnetic Resonance Imaging may be used to identify lateral medullary infarct, the diagnosis is often made based on clinical features. See above.
(b) Required to attribute a voice problem to the medical diagnosis: Hoarseness, voice weakness not wholly attributable to other causes.

Severity criteria.

(a) Medical: See Introduction

(b) Vocal: See Introduction

7315. Parkinson Disease

Essential features. This condition is characterized by bradykinesia, hypokinesia (hypometria), rigidity, and resting tremor (3–5 Hz) related to progressive loss of dopaminergic cells in the substantia nigra.

Associated features. Bowed vocal folds on nasendoscopy and increased vocal fold tension reducing the speed of vocal fold movement. Hypophonia (reduced loudness and monopitch) and more generally hypokinetic dysarthria, dysphagia, and bradykinesia are the most frequent associated features of this condition. In the case of voice and speech, patients are frequently unaware of their reduced level of loudness. They also perceive their phonatory effort as elevated. Patients exhibit a lack of facial expression.

Vocal impairment. Vocal impairment is characterized as a weak voice that can be improved with prompting. In addition, individuals exhibit monoloudness, monopitch, and their speech gives the impression of rapid rate because of reduced articulatory range of motion (hypometria), despite articulatory bradykinesia. Intelligibility is further reduced by imprecise articulation, and slow and imprecise voice onsets and offsets.

Aerodynamic characteristics: Average airflow may be increased, but this will depend upon respiratory function, which may become compromised in later stages.

Acoustic characteristics: Average fundamental frequency is within normal limits and intensity is reduced.

Age at onset. Average age of onset is 60 years. Onset before the age of 40 is relatively uncommon, but does occur particularly in familial forms.

Course. Voice and speech problems may occur early in the course of the disease and progress to pose significant obstacles to communication. Dysphagia often develops in the later stages of the disease.

Complications. Dysphagia, aspiration pneumonia, decreased mobility, loss of ability to communicate, loss of ability to take oral nutrition, and death.

Predisposing factors. 15–20% of cases are familial. Earlier onset cases are more likely to be genetic in origin. All cases involve loss of dopaminergic cells in the substantia nigra. Lewy bodies are present on autopsy.

Frequency. Affects 1% of individuals older than 60 years of age; 120 per 100,000 people are affected in the United States. Seventy percent of people with PD develop speech deficits.

Sex ratio. Parkinson Disease is 1.5 times more common in men than women.

Familial pattern. Several genetic mutations have been found in large families, some affecting the protein alpha-synuclein, in autosomal dominant parkinsonism. Another genetic defect affects the protein Parkin in autosomal recessive parkinsonism with a late onset.

Differential diagnosis. Essential Tremor, Multiple Systems Atrophy, Alzheimer's Disease, depression, Progressive Supranuclear Palsy, lacunar syndromes.

Classification criteria.

(a) Required for medical diagnosis: Two of the following three criteria must be present: 1) resting tremor, 2) rigidity, and 3) bradykinesia.

(b) Required to attribute a voice problem to the medical diagnosis: Hypokinetic dysarthria including hypophonia, not attributable to other causes.

Severity criteria.

(a) Medical: See Introduction

(b) Vocal: See Introduction

7320. Multiple Systems Atrophy (Shy-Drager Syndrome, Striatonigral Degeneration, Sporadic Olivopontocerebellar Atrophy)

Essential features. Multiple Systems Atrophy (MSA) encompasses a variety of neuropathic disorders with various predominant system failures. The American Autonomic Society and the American Academy of Neurology define MSA "as a sporadic, progressive, neurodegenerative disease of undetermined etiology, characterized by extrapyramidal, pyramidal, cerebellar, and autonomic dysfunction in any combination" (Diedrich, 2002). The predominant feature determines the specific nomenclature for the disease. Shy-Drager or MSA-A indicates a predominant feature of autonomic failure, Striatonigral Degeneration or MSA-P indicates a dominance of extrapyramidal feature, and Sporadic Olivopontocerebellar Atrophy, or MSA-C indicates a dominance of cerebellar features. Neuropathology indicates the presence of many glial cytoplasmic inclusions and the absence of Lewy bodies in MSA in general.

Associated features. MSA is characterized by some combination of parkinsonism (bradykinesia, rigidity, gait abnormality, and tremor), bilateral vocal fold paralysis, autonomic dysfunction manifesting as orthostatic hypotension, urinary and rectal incontinence, impotence, and loss of sweating. Voice and speech signs and symptoms may include laryngeal stridor, hoarseness, intermittent glottal fry, and slow speech rate. Although all of these signs and symptoms can occur in MSA, each of them is not always present and a number of other deviant speech features may be present. The voice impairment in MSA can be quite variable, depending on the specific dysarthria type that is associated with it, and may also vary across individuals. Bilateral vocal fold paralysis and dysphagia can occur in the later stages of some forms of the disease.

Vocal impairment. Vocal and speech impairment when present may be characterized by a breathy and strained voice quality, reduced loudness, monopitch and monoloudness, imprecise consonants, intermittent glottal fry, a slow and deliberate speaking rate, or variations in rate, suggesting a flaccid type of dysarthria. Limited ability to achieve precise voice offsets and onsets may also occur.

Aerodynamic characteristics: When vocal impairment is present, airflow may be increased if the vocal folds do not offer normal resistance.

Acoustic characteristics: Intensity is predicted to be reduced.

Age at onset. Typical onset is in the 5th to 6th decades.

Course. The progression of neurodegenerative symptoms result in death in approximately 6–10 years following onset. Older age at onset typically predicts shorter duration of disease prior to death. Bronchopneumonia and sudden death are common.

Complications. Bilateral vocal fold paralysis usually requires tracheostomy in the later stages of the disease. A feeding tube may be required because of swallowing problems.

Predisposing factors. Unknown.

Frequency. MSA overall: 2–15 per 100,000. It is estimated that 25,000–100,000 individuals in the United States have MSA. The disease has been found in all races.

Sex ratio. MSA overall: More males than females (3–9:1).

Familial pattern. MSA overall: Non-familial.

Differential diagnosis. Parkinson Disease (PD), Pure Autonomic Failure, Alzheimer's Disease, Huntington's Disease, multi-infarct dementia, Multiple Sclerosis, Hallervorden-Spatz disease. Differentiation of MSA and Parkinson Disease rests on the following observations: poor response to levodopa in MSA, in contrast to good response in PD; rapid progression of symptoms in MSA, in contrast to slow progression in PD; early onset of instability and falling in MSA, versus late onset of instability and falling in PD; 40% of patients with MSA are in a wheelchair within 5 years of onset in MSA, compared to a slower progressive disability in PD; Lewy bodies are absent in MSA and occur primarily in the substantia nigra in PD; cytoplasmic inclusions occur in MSA and not in PD; thermal regulation is affected in MSA and is normal in PD.

Classification criteria.

(a) Required for medical diagnosis:

MSA–A (Shy-Drager): Diagnosis by a neurologist indicates a predominance of autonomic features in the disease. Bilateral vocal fold paralysis may be present.

MSA–P: Diagnosis by a neurologist may rest upon no therapeutic response to levodopa, and presence of orthostatic hypotension, dysarthria (which may or may not be present), stridor, and, in some individuals, contractures and dystonia. These symptoms are rare in Parkinson Disease.

MSA–C: This type of MSA is characterized by gait ataxia, limb kinetic ataxia, and sometimes ataxic dysarthria.

(b) Required to attribute a voice problem to the medical diagnosis: Dysarthria, voice, or respiratory disturbance consistent with medical findings.

Severity criteria.

(a) Medical: See Introduction

(b) Vocal: See Introduction

7325. Progressive Supranuclear Palsy (PSP) (includes Pseudobulbar Palsy and Steele-Richardson-Olszewski Syndrome)

Essential features. A neurodegenerative disease of the brainstem and cerebellum with early gait instability and difficulty with normal vertical eye movement.

Associated features. Mild dementia, emotional lability, depression, irritability, and apathy. Different types of dysarthria may be present, the most common being mixed dysarthria with some combination of hypokinetic, spastic, and ataxic types. Dysphagia is also common.

Vocal Impairment. Vocal impairment varies, depending on the type of dysarthria or mixed dysarthria. Voice and speech may be hypokinetic, spastic, or ataxic with hypernasality.

Aerodynamic characteristics: Variable across patients, depending on the type of dysarthria.

Acoustic characteristics: Variable across patients, depending on the type of dysarthria.

Age at onset. Typically in the 5th to 7th decades.

Course. Characteristic early signs are gait instability and falls. Patients typically fall backwards, due to rigidity in the muscles of the back of the neck resulting in an extended spine. These observations regarding falling contrast with those for individuals with Parkinson Disease, who typically fall forward in later disease stages. Also early in PSP, patients experience abnormalities in eye movements, the first sign being difficulty looking up or down. Speech and voice problems may also be early occurring. Progression of neurodegenerative symptoms such as dysphagia may lead to death. Death typically occurs within 10 years.

Complications. Injuries related to falling; severe dysphagia resulting in aspiration pneumonia.

Predisposing factors. Unknown.

Frequency. 1.39 per 100,000.

Sex ratio. Slight male predominance (1.5:1).

Familial pattern. Non-familial.

Differential diagnosis. Parkinson Disease, Alzheimer's Disease, Huntington's Disease, multi-infarct dementia, Multiple Sclerosis, Hallervorden-Spatz disease, Multiple Systems Atrophy.

Classification criteria.

(a) Required for medical diagnosis: Diagnosis by a neurologist usually depends upon the paralysis of vertical gaze, combined with Parkinsonian symptoms (bradykinesia and rigidity) and postural instability. Unlike PD, tremor is usually absent in PSP.

(b) Required to attribute a voice problem to the medical diagnosis: Hypokinetic, spastic, and/or ataxic dysarthria characterize speech and voice.

Severity criteria.

(a) Medical criteria: See Introduction

(b) Vocal criteria: See Introduction

7330. Multiple Sclerosis (MS)

Essential features. An inflammatory demyelinating disease, which can affect multiple and disseminated sites. Sensory and motor impairments of the limbs, cognitive problems, tremor, and visual disturbances are most common. The most common presentation of MS involves alternating attacks and relapses in the early stages of disease and then progression of signs and symptoms. Motor symptoms include muscle weakness and difficulties with coordination and balance. Cognitive impairments include difficulties with concentration, attention, memory, and judgment.

Associated features. Associated features may include dysarthria, nystagmus, intention tremor, trigeminal neuralgia, Bell's palsy, and facial myokymia (rippling movements under the skin). Dysarthria may involve almost any type or combination of types. Although spastic-ataxic dysarthria may be common, it is not the only possible dysarthria type.

Vocal impairment. Voice may be affected by almost any type of dysarthria, or combination of types. Although spastic-ataxic dysarthria may be common, it is not the only possible dysarthria type.

Aerodynamic characteristics: Variable within and across patients.

Acoustic characteristics: Variable within and across patients.

Age at onset. Onset most commonly occurs between ages 18–40 years.

Course. The disease advances intermittently with periods of remission. MS can also be primarily progressive without relapses. Severe dysphagia develops and aspiration pneumonia is often the cause of death.

Complications. Pneumonia, death (life expectancy is approximately 7 years shorter in patients with MS than in the general population). Dysphagia is a significant complication later in the course of the disease.

Predisposing factors. Caucasian, living in northern regions. Genetic predisposition may be involved in some cases.

Frequency. 350,000 people have known MS in the United States; 10,000 new patients are diagnosed each year. More than 1 million people are affected worldwide.

Sex ratio. More frequent in women (1.6-2:1).

Familial pattern. There do appear to be genetic predisposing factors as illustrated in twin studies. However, the connection is poorly defined at this time.

Differential diagnosis. Essential Tremor, hemifacial spasm, Lyme disease, spinal cord infarction, metabolic disease.

Classification criteria.

(a) Required for medical diagnosis: History, physical examination, and Magnetic Resonance Imaging (MRI) findings of plaques shown as T2 hyperintensities in the periventricular regions consistent with MS.

(b) Required to attribute a voice problem to the medical diagnosis: Recurring episodes of weak, strained, or breathy voice in conjunction with disease relapse. Spastic-ataxic dysarthria is common but not exclusive.

Severity criteria.

(a) Medical: See Introduction

(b) Vocal: See Introduction

7335. Cerebellar Disorders

Essential features. Insult or disease affecting the cerebellum. A large number of syndromes may affect cerebellar function. Many are familial.

Associated features. Decreased motor coordination, which is diffuse across many systems. Ataxic speech characterized by imprecise articulation, variable rate, pitch, loudness, and stress variation. Some reports indicate intermittent hyperadduction of the vocal folds, vocal tremor, and harsh/strained voice quality. Motor learning may be impaired.

Vocal impairment. Vocal impairment may vary significantly, often involving strained vocalization with intermittent hyperadduction similar to spasmodic dysphonia. Speech rhythm and intonation patterns are abnormal, demonstrating a stereotyped quality with reduced rate of speech ("scanning speech").

Aerodynamic characteristics: Unknown.

Acoustic characteristics: Unknown.

Age at onset. Variable; dependent upon type of injury or disease process.

Course. Variable.

Complications. Vary with disease or trauma.

Predisposing factors. Familial cerebellar degeneration.

Frequency. Unknown.

Sex ratio. Unknown.

Familial pattern. Varies with disease; some forms of cerebellar disease have a genetic basis.

Differential diagnosis. Other movement disorders, acute intoxication, psychogenic voice disorder.

Classification criteria.

(a) Required for medical diagnosis: History of insult or disease affecting the cerebellum.

(b) Required to attribute a voice problem to the medical diagnosis: Voice disruption with appropriate history for cerebellar dysfunction. Presence of ataxic speech increases confidence in the attribution of the problem to cerebellar dysfunction.

Severity criteria.

(a) Medical: See Introduction

(b) Vocal: See Introduction

7340. Huntington's Chorea (HC)

Essential features. Disease involving cell loss of the basal ganglia and cortical neurons, typically characterized by adult onset and autonomic dominant inheritance. HC is also typically manifested by involuntary movements, dementia, and behavioral changes.

Associated features. Generalized impairment in motor control including poor hand, oral motor, pharyngeal, and laryngeal control due to involuntary choreic movements; dysarthria, inspiratory grunts, slow speech, hyperkinetic dysarthria, and dysphagia.

Vocal impairment. The voice of patients with HC is commonly characterized by hyperkinetic dysarthria. Pitch and loudness are uncontrolled.

Aerodynamic characteristics: Unknown.

Acoustic characteristics: Unknown.

Age at onset. Onset usually occurs after age 35. However, 10% of patients with HC have juvenile onset, with onset prior to age 20. Onset before the age of 10 and after 70 is rare.

Course. Progressive condition with eventual death due to intercurrent disease (preexisting illness). Pneumonia and cardiovascular complications are the most common cause of death. With the juvenile onset form, muscular rigidity is the most common presentation.

Complications. Pneumonia.

Predisposing factors. Presence of genetic mutation.

Frequency. In the U.S., 4.1–8.4 per 100,000. Internationally, the incidence varies greatly.

Sex ratio. Males and females are diagnosed with equal frequency.

Familial pattern. Autosomal dominant.

Differential diagnosis. Multiple Sclerosis, Systemic Lupus Erythematosus, Chorea Gravidarum, Neuroacanthocytosis.

Classification criteria.

(a) Required for medical diagnosis: Genetic testing results consistent with HC.

(b) Required to attribute a voice problem to the medical diagnosis: Hyperkinetic dysarthria, harsh voice, uncontrolled loudness or pitch bursts.

Severity criteria.

(a) Medical: See Introduction

(b) Vocal: See Introduction

7345. Bilateral Recurrent Laryngeal Nerve Paralysis–Central

Essential features. This condition is caused by centrally induced bilateral vagal pathology affecting the laryngeal motor neurons. This condition manifests as bilateral immobility of the vocal folds.

Associated features. The nature and severity of associated features are dependent on the position of the immobile vocal folds affecting the size of the glottis. The most typical feature is inspiratory stridor when the vocal folds are paralyzed in the median position. In severe cases, airway obstruction may occur during bilateral vocal fold paralysis in that position. A breathy and rough voice quality, vocal fatigue, and aspiration during swallowing may occur when the vocal folds are paralyzed in a lateral or paramedian position.

Vocal impairment. Vocal impairment is dependent on the position of the immobile vocal folds. The voice quality is breathy and rough, and pitch and loudness ranges are reduced when the vocal folds are paralyzed in a lateral or paramedian position. The voice quality is predicted to be minimally affected when the vocal folds are paralyzed in a median position.

> *Aerodynamic characteristics:* Increased airflow may occur when the vocal folds are paralyzed in a lateral or paramedian position. Airflow may approximate normal when the vocal folds are paralyzed in a median position.

> *Acoustic characteristics:* It is predicted that fundamental frequency will be normal and intensity range will be reduced.

Age at onset. This condition is more likely to occur in older age groups. For hereditary neuronopathies, paralysis may be present from birth or childhood.

Course. A common scenario for bilateral vocal fold paralysis involves initial presentation of a weak, breathy voice quality. As denervation persists, the vocal folds may come closer to the midline so that voice production is maintained, but the airway is severely compromised.

Complications. Airway obstruction or aspiration dependent on the position of the immobile vocal folds.

Predisposing factors. Causes include viral infection (e.g., encephalitis), concussion, brainstem compression (Arnold-Chiari Syndrome), brainstem infarct, neoplasms, and familial neuronopathies.

Frequency. This condition is considered rare, with an estimated 1,500 cases per year in the U.S., most of which were due to trauma.

Sex ratio. No difference between males and females.

Familial pattern. Autosomal dominant pattern of inheritance in congenital conditions.

Differential diagnosis. Psychogenic airway obstruction, paradoxical vocal fold motion; with chronic development, may involve neurodegenerative diseases such as multiple systems atrophy, amyotrophic lateral sclerosis, or hereditary neuropathies.

Classification criteria.

(a) Required for medical diagnosis: Visualization of the larynx demonstrating impaired adduction and abduction of both vocal folds during inspiration and expiration, with evidence of central nervous system involvement, and not wholly attributable to other causes.

(b) Required to attribute a voice problem to the medical diagnosis: Voice changes consistent with physical findings associated with bilateral vocal fold paralysis, not wholly attributable to other causes.

Severity criteria.

(a) Medical: See Introduction

(b) Vocal: See Introduction

7350. Myoclonus (Non-epileptic myoclonus, physiologic myoclonus, palatal myoclonus, diaphragmatic flutter, myoclonus velopharyngo-laryngo-oculo-diaphragmatiques)

Essential features. This condition is characterized by sudden, brief, involuntary muscle jerks typically indicative of damage to the central nervous system. Myoclonic jerks may also occur in isolation (e.g., hiccup). Myoclonic activity may present as a sequence of jerks either with or without a pattern. Onset of this condition is most frequently noted when individuals initiate a movement rather than during resting or sleep. However, spontaneous myoclonus can occur. In children, this condition is triggered by startle reflexes, sensory stimulation, or upon initiation of movement. The four classification categories of myoclonus include physiologic, essential, epileptic, and symptomatic. Physiologic myoclonus occurs in neurologically normal individuals and is diagnosed by patient report (e.g., sudden jerking during sleep). Essential myoclonus indicates idiopathic onset of this condition as the prominent problem. Epileptic myoclonus occurs in individuals with chronic seizure disorders and may be the primary component of the seizure, or occur in combination with other forms of seizure. Symptomatic myoclonus is the most common form of this condition associated with neurologic disease, post-infectious or infectious diseases, drugs, toxins, metabolic diseases, hypoxia, or neoplastic etiologies. Myoclonus evidenced through voice production may result from the presence of this condition in the muscles of the respiratory, laryngeal, or articulatory structures.

Associated features. This condition is categorized according to the areas of the body affected, electrophysiologic patterns, and the area of the central nervous system affected. This condition is typically associated with such disorders as multiple sclerosis, Parkinson disease, Alzheimer's disease, and Creutzfeldt-Jakob disease. It can also result from hypoxia or metabolic encephalopathy. Electrophysiology is used to determine whether the source of the myoclonus originates from the cortex, subcortical structures, or from the spinal cord. *Prolonged hiccups* are a form of physiologic myoclonus resulting from bursts of muscle activity in the diaphragm and external intercostal muscles, resulting in sudden inhalation and possibly inhalation phonation. *Palatal myoclonus* is characterized by rhythmic involuntary elevation of the soft palate that may be viewed as a tremor in this structure. Palatal muscles associated with elevation will exhibit bursts of activity at a rate of 2 Hz. The latter is often associated with brainstem lesions, but may also be considered a benign essential palatal myoclonus. These individuals may complain of a rhythmic clicking sound in their ears. *Myoclonus velopharyngo-laryngo-oculo-diaphragmatiques* is characterized by complex and synchronous rhythmic movements in the diaphragm, shoulder, neck, arm, pharynx, larynx, eyes, and face. *Diaphragmatic flutter* is characterized by bilateral rhythmic contractions of the diaphragm muscle at rates varying from 60–200 Hz resulting in involuntary abdominal movements. These individuals may complain of sudden involuntary inhalation during speech. A common complaint of patients with myoclonus affecting the speech mechanism is impaired intelligibility. Myoclonus causing sudden involuntary contractions of the intrinsic muscles of the larynx can disrupt connected speech and may be associated with aspiration during swallowing due to sudden opening of the larynx in the presence of a bolus of food.

Vocal impairment. Vocal impairment will depend on the affected structures in the speech mechanism. *Prolonged hiccups* are a form of physiologic myoclonus resulting from bursts of muscle activity in the diaphragm and external intercostal muscles, resulting in sudden inhalation and possibly inhalation phonation. *Palatal myoclonus* is characterized by rhythmic involuntary elevation of the soft palate that may be viewed as a tremor in this structure. Palatal muscles associated with elevation will exhibit bursts of activity at a rate of 2 Hz. The latter is often associated with brainstem lesions, but may also be considered a benign essential palatal myoclonus. These individuals may complain of a rhythmic clicking sound in their ears. *Myoclonus velopharyngo-laryngo-oculo-diaphragmatiques* is characterized by complex and synchronous rhythmic movements in the diaphragm, shoulder, neck, arm, pharynx, larynx, eyes, and face. *Diaphragmatic flutter* is characterized by bilateral rhythmic contractions of the diaphragm muscle at rates varying from 60–200 Hz resulting in involuntary abdominal movements. These individuals may complain of sudden involuntary inhalation during speech. Myoclonus causing sudden involuntary contractions of the intrinsic muscles of the larynx can disrupt connected speech and may be associated with aspiration during swallowing due to sudden opening of the larynx in the presence of a bolus of food.

Aerodynamic characteristics: Unknown.

Acoustic characteristics: Unknown.

Age at onset. Variable, but most commonly seen in adulthood.

Course. Onset of this condition frequently occurs subsequent to lesions of the cortical or subcortical structures and spinal cord. It may also arise spontaneously with prolongation of normal myoclonic contractions such as with hiccups.

Complications. Difficulty moving adequately to perform daily activities of living such as standing, walking, grasping objects, eating, writing, or speaking.

Predisposing factors. Lesions in the central nervous system, hypoxia, metabolic encephalopathy.

Frequency. Unknown.

Sex ratio. Unknown.

Familial pattern. Unknown.

Differential diagnosis. Seizure disorders, tics, essential tremor, dystonic tremor, psychogenic tremor, psychogenic myoclonus, hereditary, metabolic, mitochondrial, infectious, vascular, neoplastic, toxic, or neurodegenerative disease processes.

Classification criteria.

(a) Required for medical diagnosis: Evidence of sudden, brief, muscle jerks in response to initiation of movement, exacerbated startle response, or sensory stimulation, frequently subsequent to a known central nervous system lesion affecting the cortex, subcortical structures, or spinal cord. Thorough characterization would include a description of the degree of involvement of structures (e.g., focal versus generalized), the pattern of involvement (e.g., intermittent versus continuous), and the means of triggering the condition (e.g., present at rest, during initiation of movement, or as part of a startle response).

(b) Required to attribute a voice problem to the medical diagnosis: Same as for medical diagnosis.

Severity criteria.

(a) Medical: See Introduction.

(b) Vocal: See Introduction.

8000. OTHER DISORDERS AFFECTING VOICE

8010. Muscle Tension Dysphonia (Primary) (Hyperfunctional voice disorder, hypoadducted hyperfunction, etc.)

Essential features. Dysphonia in the *absence* of current organic vocal fold pathology, without obvious psychogenic or neurologic etiology, associated with excessive, atypical or abnormal laryngeal movements during phonation. Observations during rigid or flexible laryngoscopy may reveal consistent laryngeal or supraglottic constriction or vocal fold hypoadduction during phonation. However, visual evidence of hyper- and hypoadduction or anteroposterior constriction must be interpreted within the context of other clinical evidence (e.g., patient response to scoping, case history report, voice probes, etc.). Although abnormal muscle tension has been presumed clinically (hence, the prevalence of the term "Muscle Tension Dysphonia"), few objective studies have substantiated abnormal muscular tensions empirically. The classification Muscle Tension Dysphonia represents a persistent, unexplained dysphonia that is behaviorally modifiable.

Associated features. Pain on phonation or swallowing and vocal fatigue may be reported.

Vocal impairment. Vocal impairment may vary. In some cases, voice quality may be normal or near normal with the primary complaint being vocal fatigue and/or odynophonia. Various aberrant laryngeal postures or movements indicating hyperfunction or other atypical vocal behaviors may be observed. False fold constriction with or without arytenoid-epiglottis approximation is common. Also, vocal fold hypoadduction is commonly reported. In addition, postural abnormalities of the true vocal folds may be observed during phonation. Behaviors identified as aberrant may not always be associated with excessive muscle tension.

Aerodynamic characteristics: Variable within and across cases.

Acoustic characteristics: Variable within and across cases.

Age at onset. Variable, but most commonly seen in adulthood.

Course. A disorder that may fluctuate in severity but may not fully remit without intervention. Sudden onset may occur following an acute episode of upper respiratory tract infection or laryngitis associated with various etiologies, including irritation of laryngeal structures by bacterial, viral, chemical, or thermal stimuli, with persistence of voice dysfunction following resolution of the laryngitis.

Complications. Some clinicians suggest that phonotraumatic lesions are one potential sequela of long-standing Muscle Tension Dysphonia (Primary). Social and occupational limitations may be present.

Predisposing factors. Precipitating event or events, possibly unrecognized and/or already resolved, that cause(s) a change in the usual manner of voice production. Introverted personality may be a factor (Roy & Bless, 2000a; 2000b).

Frequency. Unknown.

Sex ratio. Unknown, although more females than males seek treatment for this disorder.

Familial pattern. Unknown.

Differential diagnosis. Muscle Tension/Adaptive Dysphonia Secondary (8020), structural, neurologic (including spasmodic dysphonia), or psychogenic source of dysphonia.

Classification criteria.

(a) Required for medical diagnosis: Evidence of excessive or atypical laryngeal movements, or postures affecting phonation without identifiable cause.

(b) Required to attribute a voice problem to the medical diagnosis: Same as for medical diagnosis.

Severity criteria. As noted, a variety of laryngeal movements and postures are associated with Muscle Tension Dysphonia (Primary). False fold constriction and arytenoids to epiglottis approximation are frequently noted, but other gestures may also be observed. Severity depends on specifics of voice production and resulting voice quality.

(a) Medical: See Introduction

(b) Vocal: See Introduction

8020. Muscle Tension/Adaptive Dysphonia (Secondary)
(Hyperfunctional voice disorder, hypoadducted
hyperfunction, etc.)

Essential features. Dysphonia in the *presence* of current organic vocal fold pathology, psychogenic, or neurologic etiology, originating
as a compensatory response to the primary etiology. The resulting
dysphonia may include excessive or atypical laryngeal movements
during phonation. Observations with rigid or flexible endoscopy may
reveal consistent laryngeal or supraglottic constriction during
phonation, as visualized during rigid or flexible laryngoscopy. The
term "adaptive" is added here to reflect an alteration in the normal or
usual manner of phonation in response to glottal incompetence or
other organic pathology.

Associated features. Pain on phonation, pain during swallowing, or
vocal fatigue.

Vocal impairment. Vocal impairment may vary. In some cases, voice
quality may be normal or near normal with the primary complaint being vocal fatigue or odynophonia. In other cases, voice abnormality
may be related mostly to the underlying condition. A variety of aberrant vocal behaviors may be observed.

Aerodynamic characteristics: Variable within and across cases.

Acoustic characteristics: Variable within and across cases.

Age at onset. Variable, but most commonly seen in adulthood.

Course. The condition is likely associated with onset of glottal incompetence or other pathology that affects normal phonation/vocal fold vibration.

Complications. Phonotraumatic lesions may result from Muscle Ten-
sion/Adaptive Dysphonia (Secondary), thereby intensifying the condition. Social and occupational limitations may occur.

Predisposing factors. Glottal incompetence of any origin (lesions, scar, paralysis, loss of true vocal fold tissue due to ablation from cancer surgery, etc.); irritants to the airway (e.g., chemical, smoke, or dust exposure); other organic pathology that impedes phonation/vocal fold vibration. Extroverted personality with an inability to inhibit may be a factor (Roy & Bless, 2000 a, b).

Frequency. Unknown.

Sex ratio. Unknown.

Familial pattern. Unknown.

Differential diagnosis. Muscle Tension Dysphonia Primary (8010), psychogenic dysphonia.

Classification criteria.

(a) Required for medical diagnosis: Evidence of excessive or atypical laryngeal activity in conjunction with glottal incompetence or other laryngeal pathology, as visualized by flexible and/or rigid endoscopy. False vocal fold constriction with or without arytenoid-epiglottic approximation are common.

(b) Required to attribute a voice problem to the medical diagnosis: Hoarseness, odynophonia, and vocal fatigue, not wholly attributable to other causes.

Severity criteria. As noted, a variety of laryngeal movements and postures are associated with Muscle Tension/Adaptive Dysphonia (Secondary). False fold constriction and arytenoids to epiglottis approximation are frequently noted.

(a) Medical: See Introduction

(b) Vocal: See Introduction

8030. Ventricular Dysphonia

Essential features. Dysphonia in which vocalization is produced by vibration of the false vocal folds, typically in association with approximation of the false vocal folds.

Associated features. Low-pitched, raspy voice due to relatively large oscillatory mass of the false vocal folds as vibratory structures. Most commonly, ventricular phonation is a compensatory behavior used to produce an alternative sound source in response to limitations in true vocal fold vibration. Less commonly, vibration of the arytenoid complex and epiglottic tip has been observed as an secondary compensatory gesture, when true vocal fold vibration is impaired. Ventricular phonation may also be present in conjunction with true vocal fold phonation.

Vocal impairment. Ventricular phonation is characterized by both low intensity and low frequency, often with pronounced roughness. The voice is often difficult to hear with any kind of background noise. Other characteristic findings include the limitations in pitch range and flexibility, limited vocal endurance, and rapid fatigue and pain due to increased effort required for phonation.

Aerodynamic characteristics: Variable.

Acoustic characteristics: Low fundamental frequency is characteristic. Reduced frequency and intensity ranges are likely.

Age at onset. May occur in young children in association with significant laryngeal pathology, such as scarred vocal folds due to numerous surgical excisions of papilloma. May also occur at any age as a compensatory behavior due to dysfunction of the true vocal folds or as a manifestation of Muscle Tension/Adaptive Dysphonia (Secondary) (8020) due to psychogenic etiology.

Course. Variable, partly depending on co-occurring laryngeal status.

Complications. Severe hypertrophy of ventricular folds.

Predisposing factors. Conditions that result in glottal incompetence and impairment of true vocal fold vibration.

Frequency. Unknown.

Sex ratio. Unknown.

Familial pattern. No familial pattern has been observed.

Differential diagnosis. Conditions that impair true vocal fold mobility, psychogenic dysphonia. If phonatory false vocal fold vibration is confirmed, competing diagnoses do not exist. However, identification of the underlying causal etiology is critical.

Classification criteria.

(a) Required for medical diagnosis: Ventricular fold approximation that results in observable vibratory behavior of the ventricular folds, with or without confirmed true vocal fold vibration. These observations are made through laryngeal imaging.

(b) Required to attribute a voice problem to the medical diagnosis: Low, raspy voice consistent with false vocal fold phonation.

Severity criteria.

(a) Medical: See Introduction

(b) Vocal: See Introduction

8040. Paradoxical Vocal Fold Movement Disorder (Vocal Cord Dysfunction) (PVFMD)

Essential features. Demonstrable episodes of vocal fold adduction, possibly associated with non-communicative phonation, during inspiration, expiration (less commonly), or both. Inspiratory volumes in the flow-volume loop are characteristically reduced, whereas expiratory volumes are normal during episodes.

Associated features. Respiratory distress, cough, globus sensation, dysphonia, stridor, hypersensitivity to various agents, shortness of breath with or without exertion. PVFMD co-occurs with asthma in approximately 50% of patients, but unfortunately, isolated PVFMD is often misdiagnosed and treated inappropriately as asthma.

Vocal impairment. Dysphonia, if present, is not due to the paradoxical motion of the vocal folds, but may be an associated feature.

Age at onset. Variable; depending upon which etiologic factor is associated with the PVFMD. Documented age range is 4 months to 83 years of age.

Course. This can be a chronic condition or may involve acute episodes. Symptoms may range from mild respiratory annoyance to severe respiratory distress requiring hospitalization.

Complications. Significant complications associated with PVFMD may be medical and psychosocial. Although as many as 50% of patients with PVFMD also have confirmed diagnoses of asthma, this frequent combination has complicated the diagnosis for patients without asthma, who may have been treated inappropriately with subsequent negative sequelae (steroid treatments, tracheostomy, or endotracheal intubation).

Predisposing factors. Predisposing factors are numerous. Some common factors include asthma, exposure to environmental pollutants or allergens, stress, and athletic exertion, in susceptible individuals. Laryngopharyngeal reflux disease, neurologic factors (e.g., vagal disorder, vocal fold paresis, Arnold-Chiari Malformation), chemical sensitivity, structural abnormality (e.g., laryngomalacia), or psychogenic factors may predispose individuals to PVFMD. In some cases, the condition may represent poor management of air exchange in the face of extreme pulmonary demands, as with athletics. For example, breathing rates may be increased, with decreased inspiratory volumes and normal expiratory volumes.

Frequency. PVFMD is found in 10–15% of patients seeking care for asthma. However, PVFMD and asthma can, and often do, co-exist. Inspiratory stridor may occur in up to 5% of elite athletes.

Sex ratio. Appears to be more prevalent in females (approximately 7:3) in adolescence.

Familial pattern. Unknown.

Differential diagnosis. Asthma (PVFMD will be unresponsive to methylcholine challenge), foreign body obstruction, bilateral vocal fold paralysis, chronic obstructive pulmonary disease, Reinke's edema, anaphylaxis, LPR, vocal fold spasms.

Classification criteria.

(a) Required for medical diagnosis: Observed vocal fold adduction during inspiration, with or without exposure to triggers and with the appropriate history. For some patients, symptoms of glottic narrowing occur during expiration as well.

(b) Required to attribute a voice problem to the medical diagnosis: Not relevant.

Severity criteria.

(a) Medical: See Introduction

(b) Vocal : See Introduction

9000. VOICE DISORDERS: UNDIAGNOSED OR NOT OTHERWISE SPECIFIED (NOS)

This category is appropriate for those cases that do not satisfy the classification criteria described in this text. It may be that the clinician is unable to determine the source of dysphonia, or that the classification criteria may not be met in totality, or that a suspected diagnosis is pending. Thus, this category may be used for patients with complaints of significant and consistent voice changes, or dysphonia that cannot be explained by a medical condition or substance use, and who do not meet criteria for other conditions described in this text.

REFERENCES

Adametz, J. and J. L. O'Leary (1959). "Experimental mutism resulting from periaqueductal lesions in cats." *Neurol. Minneap.* **9**: 636–642.

Adams, J. A. and L. E. Hufford (1962). "Contributions of a part-task trainer to the learning and relearning of a time-shared flight maneuver." *Human Factors* **4**: 159–170.

Adams, J. A. (1987). "Historical review and appraisal of research on the learning, retention and transfer of human motor skills." *Psychological Bulletin* **101**: 41–74.

Aidley, D. J. (1998). *The physiology of excitable cells*. Cambridge, UK: Cambridge University Press.

AJCC (American Joint Committee on Cancer) Cancer Staging Manual, Sixth Edition, American Joint Committee on Cancer; Springer-Verlag New York: 2002.

Akbayir, N., Basak, T., Seven, H., Sungun, A., & Erdem, L. (2004). Investigation of Helicobacter pylori colonization in laryngeal neoplasia. *Eur Arch Otorhinolaryngolo,* **30**.

Akhtar, S., G. Wood, et al. (1999). "Effect of caffeine on the vocal folds: a pilot study." *J Laryngol Otol* **113**(4): 341–5.

al-Shammari, S. A., T. Khoja, et al. (1995). "Compliance with short-term antibiotic therapy among patients attending primary health centres in Riyadh, Saudi Arabia." *J R Soc Health* **115**(4): 231–4.

Alewijnse, D., I. Mesters, et al. (2001). "Predictors of intention to adhere to physiotherapy among women with urinary incontinence." *Health Educ Res* **16**(2): 173–86.

Ammons, R. B. (1950). "Acquisition of motor skill: III. Effects of initially distributed practice on rotary pursuit performance." *Journal of Experimental Psychology* **40**: 777–787.

Aronson, A. E. (1990). *Clinical voice disorders: An interdisciplinary approach.* New York: Thieme Stratton.

Aronson, S. C. (2002). Depression, eMedicine. **2002**.

Arsura, E. L., W. B. Kilgore, et al. (2002). Coccidiomycosis (infectious disease), eMedicine. **2002**.

Arthur, G. K. and K. Monnell (2002). Body dysmorphic disorder, eMedicine. **2002**.

Ashworth, N. L. (2002). Carpal tunnel syndrome, eMedicine. **2002**.

Association, A. P. (1994). *Diagnostic and statistical manual of mental disorders.* Washington, DC: Author.

Association, N. S. D. (nd.). Spasmodic dysphonia: symptoms, NSDA. **2002**.

Atis, S., B. Tutluoglu, et al. (2001). "Characteristics and compliance of patients receiving long-term oxygen therapy (LTOT) in Turkey." *Monaldi Arch Chest Dis* **56**(2): 105–9.

Austin, S. F. and I. R. Titze (1997). "The effect of subglottal resonance upon vocal fold vibration." *J Voice* **11**th(4th): 391–402.

Aylward, G. P., A. Lazzara, et al. (1978). "Behavioral and neurological characteristics of a hyranencephalic infant." *Developmental medicine and child neurology* **20**: 211–217.

Bacciu, A., G. Mercante, et al. (2003). "Reflux esophagitis as a possible risk factor in the development of pharyngolaryngeal squamous cell carcinoma." *Tumori* **89**(5): 485–487.

Bailey, e. a. (nd.). Laryngeal manifestations of AIDS, Head and neck surgery—Otolaryngology. **2002**.

Bajracharya, H. and D. Hinthorn (2002). Sinusitis, chronic, eMedicine. **2002**.

Baken, R. J. (1987). *Clinical measurement of speech and voice.* Boston: College-Hill Press.

Ballenger, J. J. (1977). *Diseases of the nose, throat and ear.* London: Henry Kimpton Publishers.

Bandura, A. (2002). "Self-efficacy: Toward a unifying theory of behavioral change." *Perceptual Motor Skills* **94**(3 pt. 1): 1056.

Bastian, R. W. and V. L. Lawrence (1984). "Hoarseness in singers." *NATS Bulletin* **40**(3): 26–27.

Bastian, R. W., K. Verdolini-Marston, et al. (1989). "The team approach to management of patients with voice disorders." *The NATS Journal* **45**(5): 16–19.

Baum, A., R. J. Gatchel, et al. (1983). "Emotional, behavioral, and physiological effects of chronic stress at Three Mile Island." *J Consult Clin Psychol* **51**(4): 565–72.

Belafsky, P. C., G. N. Postma, et al. (2001). "The validity and reliability of the reflux finding score (RFS)." *Laryngoscope* **111**(8): 1313–1317.

Belafsky P. C., Postma, G. N., & Koufman, J. A. (2002). Validity and reliability of the reflux symptom index (RSI). *J Voice*. **16**(2):274–7.

Ben-Sira, Z. (1980). "Affective and instrumental components in the physician–patient relationship: An additional dimension of interaction theory." *J Health Soc Behav* **21**(2): 170–80.

Bernstein, B. E. (2002). Anxiety disorder: Social phobia and selective mutism, eMedicine. **2002**.

Berry, D. A., K. Verdolini, et al. (2001). "A quantitative output–cost ratio in voice production." *Journal of Speech, Language, and Hearing Research* **44**(1): 29–37.

Bienenfeld, D. (2002). Malingering, eMedicine. **2002**.

Bilodeau, E. A., I. M. Bilodeau, et al. (1959). "Some effects of introducing and withdrawing knowledge of results early and late in practice." *Journal of Experimental Psychology* **58**: 142–144.

Bizzi, E. (1974). "The coordination of eye-head movements." *Scientific American* **231**(4): 100–106.

Black, K. J. (2002). Tourette syndrome and other tic disorders, eMedicine. **2002**.

Blalock, S. J., B. M. DeVellis, et al. (2002). "Effects of an osteoporosis prevention program incorporating tailored educational materials." *Am J Health Promot* **16**(3): 146–56.

Blitzer, A., M. F. Brin, et al. (1998). Clinical and laboratory characteristics of focal laryngeal dystonia: Study of 110 cases, PubMed. **2003**.

Bliznikas, D. and S. Baredes (2002). Spasmodic dysphonia, eMedicine. **2003**.

Boone, D. R. and S. C. McFarlane (1994). *The voice and voice therapy*. Englewood Cliffs, NJ: Prentice Hall.

Bradley, M. (1980). "Prevention and correction of vocal disorders in singers." *NATS Bulletin* **36**(5): 38–41.

Brandon, C. A., C. Rosen, et al. (2003). "Staining of human thyroarytenoid muscle with myosin antibodies reveals some unique extrafusal fibers, but no muscle spindles." *Journal of Voice* **17**(2): 245–254.

Brasic, J. R. and B. Bronson (2002). Tardive dyskinesia, eMedicine. **2002**.

Brin, M. F., Fahn, S., Blitzer, A., Ramig, L. O., & Stewart, C. (1992). Movement disorders of the larynx. In: Neurologic Disorders of the Larynx (Blitzer, A., Brin, M. F., Sasaki, C. T., Fahn, S., & Harris, K. S., Eds.). Thieme Medical Publishers, Inc.: New York, pp 248–278.

Brook, M. G., A. Dale, et al. (2001). "Adherence to highly active antiretroviral therapy in the real world: Experience of twelve English HIV units." *AIDS Patient Care STDS* **15**(9): 491–4.

Bryan, W. L. and N. Harter (1897). "Studies in the physiology and psychology of the telegraphic language." *Psychological Review* **4**: 27–53.

Bryant, N. J., G. E. Woodson, et al. (1996). "Human posterior cricoarytenoid muscle compartments: Anatomy and mechanics." *Archives of Otolaryngology—Head and Neck Surgery* **122**(12): 1331–1336.

Buddiga, P. and M. O'Connell (2002). Vocal cord dysfunction, eMedicine. **2002**.

Butler, J. E., T. H. Hammond, et al. (2001). "Gender-related differences of hyaluronic acid distribution in the human vocal fold." *Laryngoscope* **111**(5): 907–911.

Cardoso, F. and J. Jankovic (1997). Dystonia and dyskinesia, Movement Disorders Clinic, Department of Neurology, Federal University of Minas. **2003**.

Catten, M., S. Gray, et al. (1998). "Analysis of cellular location and concentration in vocal fold lamina propria." *Otolaryngology—Head and Neck Surgery* **118**(5): 663–667.

Ceccolini, E. and R. A. Schwartz (2002). Ehlers-danlos syndrome, eMedicine. **2002**.

Chang, R. C., I. Susanto, et al. (2001). Histoplasmosis, eMedicine. **2002**.

Chen, H. (2002). Marfan syndrome, eMedicine. **2002**.

Chesney, M. A., J. R. Ickovics, et al. (2000). "Self-reported adherence to antiretroviral medications among participants in HIV clinical trials: the AACTG adherence instruments. Patient Care Committee & Adherence Working Group of the Outcomes Committee of the Adult AIDS Clinical Trials Group (AACTG)." *AIDS Care* **12**(3): 255–66.

Churchill's medical dictionary. (1989). New York: Churchill Livingstone.

Cole, K. J. and J. H. Abbs (1983). "Intentional responses to kinesthetic stimuli in orofacial muscles: Implications for the coordination of speech movements." *Journal of Neuroscience* **3**(12): 2660–2669.

Colton, R. and J. K. Casper (1996). *Understanding voice problems: A physiological perspective for diagnosis and treatment.* Baltimore, MD: Williams & Wilkins.

Connor, G. S., Ondo, W.G., & Stacy, M. A. Essential Tremor: A Practical Guide to Evaluation, Diagnosis, and Treatment. Clinician (Ed. Jankovic, J.). June 2001. 19(2): 1–20.

Coyle, E. F. (1999). "Physiological determinants of endurance exercise performance." *Journal of Science and Medicine in Sport / Sports Medicine Australia* **2**(3): 181–189.

Craig, S. (2003). Hyponatremia, http://www.emedicine.com/emerg/topic275.htm.

Dalvi, A. and S. M. Bloomfield (2002). Parkinson-plus syndromes, eMedicine. **2002**.

Dangond, F. (2002). Amyotrophic lateral sclerosis, eMedicine. **2002**.

Dardaine, V., M. Ferry, et al. (1999). "[Subcutaneous perfusion of hypodermoclysis: A useful rehydration method in geriatrics]." *La Presse Medicale* **28**(40): 2246–50.

Darley, F. L., Aronson, A., & Brown, J. (1969). Differential diagnostic patterns in dysarthria. *Journal of Speech and Hearing Research, 12*, 246–296.

Davenport, W. G. and S. Pandit (2004). Dehydration in children. *Children's Health*. S. C. Gabaeff, F. Talavera and S. L. Bernstein. **2004**.

Davidoff, T. Q., M. Cunningham, et al. (2002). Sinusitis, acute, eMedicine. **2002**.

de Klerk, E. (2001). "Patient compliance with enteric-coated weekly fluoxetine during continuation treatment of major depressive disorder." *J Clin Psychiatry* **62** **Suppl 22**: 43–7.

Demirici, C. S. and W. Abuhammour (2002). Diphtheria, eMedicine. **2002**.

Derkay, C. S., Malis, D. J., Zalzal, G., Wiatrak, B. J., Kashima, H. K., & Coltrera, M. D. (1998). A staging system for assessing severity of disease and response to therapy in recurrent respiratory papillomatosis. *Laryngoscope*. Jun **108**(6): 935–937.

Deuschl, G., B. Koster, et al. (1998). "Diagnostic and pathophysiological aspects of psychogenic tremor." *Mov Disord* **13**(2): 294–302.

Deuschl, G., & Lorenz, D. Essential Tremor. Orphanet Encyclopedia. December 2003. http://www.orpha.net/data/patho/GB/uk-essentialtremor.pdf.

Deuschl, G., Raethjen, J., Lindemann, M., & Krack, P. (2001). "The pathophysiology of tremor." *Muscle Nerve, 24*: 716–735.

Diedrich, A. and D. Robertson (2002). Multiple system atrophy, eMedicine. **2002**.

DiMatteo, M. R. (1995). "Patient adherence to pharmacotherapy: The importance of effective communication." *Formulary* **30**(10): 596–8, 601–2, 605.

Disease, W. F. o. N. S. o. M. N. (1994). "El Escorial World Neurology criteria for the diagnosis of amyotrophic lateral sclerosis." *J Neurol Sci* **124**: 107.

Donohoe, G., N. Owens, et al. (2001). "Predictors of compliance with neuroleptic medication among inpatients with schizophrenia: A discriminant function analysis." *Eur Psychiatry* **16**(5): 293–8.

Dornelas, E. A., R. A. Sampson, et al. (2000). "A randomized controlled trial of smoking cessation counseling after myocardial infarction." *Prev Med* **30**(4): 261–8.

Dromey, C., Warrick, P., & Irish, J. (2002). "The influence of pitch and loudness changes on the acoustics of vocal tremor." *Journal of Speech Language Hearing Research,* **45**(5): 879–90.

Dufel, S. (2001). Conversion disorder, eMedicine. **2002**.

Duffy, E. (1962). *Activation and behavior.* New York: Wiley.

Duffy, J. R. (1995). *Motor speech disorders: Substrates, differential diagnosis, and management.* St. Louis, MO: Mosby Yearbook.

Durham, B. A. (2002). Croup, eMedicine. **2002**.

Duval, C., Panisset, M., & Sadikot, A.F. (2001). The relationship between physiological tremor and the performance of rapid alternating movements in healthy elderly subjects. Exp Brain Res, 139:412–418.

Eaker, S., H. O. Adami, et al. (2001). "Reasons women do not attend screening for cervical cancer: A population-based study in Sweden." *Prev Med* **32**(6): 482–91.

Eggenberger, E. R. and Z. F. Vanek (2002). Progressive supranuclear palsy, eMedicine. **2002**.

El-Twal, M. S. (2004). Hyponatremia, http://www.emedicine.com/med/topic1130.htm.

Eldridge, R. S. (1970). "The torsion dystonias: Literature review and genetic and clinical studies." *Neurology* **20**: 1–78.

Elwyn, T. S. and I. Ahmed (2002). Factitious disorder, eMedicine. **2002**.

Epstein, S. (1994). "Integration of the cognitive and the psychodynamic unconscious." *American Psychologist* **49**(8): 709–724.

Ernster, J. A. (2002). Vocal fold paralysis, bilateral, eMedicine. **2002**.

Eslinger, P. J. and A. R. Damasio (1986). "Preserved motor learning in Alzheimer's disease: Implications for anatomy and behavior." *The Journal of Neuroscience* **6**(10): 3006–3009.

Evangelista, L. S., J. Berg, et al. (2001). "Relationship between psychosocial variables and compliance in patients with heart failure." *Heart Lung* **30**(4): 294–301.

Finkelstein, J., G. O'Connor, et al. (2001). "Development and implementation of the home asthma telemonitoring (HAT) system to facilitate asthma self-care." *Medinfo* **10**(Pt 1): 810–4.

Fisher, K. V., J. Ligon, et al. (2001). "Phonatory effects of body fluid removal." *Journal of Speech, Language, and Hearing Research* **44**: 354–367.

Fitzmaurice, C. (1997). Breathing is meaning. *The Vocal Vision: Views on Voice.* M. Hampton and B. Acker. New York: Applause Books: 247–252.

Ford, C. N., K. Inagi, et al. (1996). "Sulcus vocalis: a rational analytical approach to diagnosis and management." *Ann Otol Rhinol Laryngol* **105**(3): 189–200.

Foster, P. and S. Hudson (1998). "From compliance to concordance: a challenge for contraceptive prescribers." *Health Care Anal* **6**(2): 123–30.

Fried, M. P. (1996). *The larynx: A multidisciplinary approach.* St. Louis, MO: Mosby-Year Book, Inc.

Garnett, J. D. (2002). Subglottic stenosis in adults, eMedicine. **2002**.

Gauffin, J. and J. Sundberg (1989). "Spectral correlates of glottal voice source waveform characteristics." *Journal of Speech and Hearing Research* **32**(3): 556–565.

Gibbs, S. R. and A. Blitzer (2000). Voice disorders and phonosurgery I, Otolaryngologic Clinics of North America. **2002**.

Gordillo, V., J. del Amo, et al. (1999). "Sociodemographic and psychological variables influencing adherence to antiretroviral therapy." *AIDS* **13**(13): 1763–9.

Gordis, L., M. Markowitz, et al. (1969). "Why patients don't follow medical advice: A study of children on long-term antistreptococcal prophylaxis." *J Pediatr* **75**(6): 957–68.

Gore, T. A. and G. Richards (2002). Posttraumatic stress disorder, eMedicine. **2002**.

Graf, P. and D. L. Schacter (1985). "Implicit and explicit memory for new associations in normal and amnesic subjects." *Journal of Experimental Psychology: Learning, Memory, and Cognition* **11**(3): 501–518.

Gray, S. D., M. Hirano, et al. (1993). Molecular and cellular structure of vocal fold tissue. *Vocal Fold Physiology: Frontiers in Basic Science*. I. R. Titze. San Diego, CA: Singular: 1–35.

Gray, S. D., S. S. Pignatari, et al. (1994). "Morphologic ultrastructure of anchoring fibers in normal vocal fold basement membrane zone." *Journal of Voice* **8**(1): 48–52.

Gray, S. D., E. Hammond, et al. (1995). "Benign pathologic responses of the larynx." *Annals of Otology, Rhinology, and Laryngology* **104**(1): 12–18.

Gray, S. D., I. R. Titze, et al. (1999). "Vocal fold proteoglycans and their influence on biomechanics." *Laryngoscope* **109**(6): 845–854.

Gray, S. D. (2000). "Cellular physiology of the vocal folds." *Otolaryngologic clinics of North America* **33**(4): 679–698.

Gray, S. D., I. R. Titze, et al. (2000). "Biomechanical and histologic observations of vocal fold fibrous proteins." *Annals of Otology, Rhinology, and Laryngology* **109**(1): 77–85.

Greene F. L., Page D. L. , Fleming I. D., et al., eds. AJCC Cancer Staging Manual. 6th ed. New York: Springer-Verlag; 2002.

Greenwald, D. and W. Stadelmann (2002). Gender reassignment, eMedicine. **2002**.

Grigsby, D. G. (2002). Malnutrition, eMedicine. **2002**.

Hacker, M. R., S. Geraghty, et al. (2001). "Barriers to compliance with prophylaxis therapy in haemophilia." *Haemophilia* **7**(4): 392–6.

Haim, D. Y., M. L. Lippmann, et al. (1995). "The pulmonary complications of crack cocaine. A comprehensive review." *Chest* **107**(1): 233–40.

Haken, H. (1977). *Synergetics: An introduction.* Heidelberg, Germany: Springer-Verlag.

Haken, H. (1983). *Advanced synergetics.* Heidelberg, Germany: Springer-Verlag.

Hamilton, J. C. and M. D. Feldman (2002). Munchausen syndrome, eMedicine. **2002**.

Hammond, T. H., Z. Ruixia, et al. (1997). "The intermediate layer: a morphologic study of the elastin and hyaluronic acid constituents of normal human vocal folds." *The Journal of Voice* **11**(1): 59–66.

Hammond, T. H., S. D. Gray, et al. (2000). "Age- and gender-related collagen distribution in human vocal folds." *Annals of Otology, Rhinology, and Laryngology* **109**(10 Pt. 1): 913–920.

Haraldson, S. J. and B. J. Blasko (2002). Repetitive motion injuries, eMedicine. **2002**.

Haria, D. M. and M. O. Salifu (2001). Chronic fatigue syndrome, eMedicine. **2002**.

Hauser, R. A. and R. Pahwa (2002). Parkinson, eMedicine. **2002**.

Heatley, D. G. and Swift, E. (1996). "Paradoxical vocal cord dysfunction in an infant with stridor and gastroesophageal reflux." *International Journal of Pediatric Otorhinolaryngology,* **34,** 149–151.

Hemler, R. J., G. H. Wieneke, et al. (1997). "The effect of relative humidity of inhaled air on acoustic parameters of voice in normal subjects." *Journal of Voice* **11**(3): 293–300.

Hemler, R. J., G. H. Wieneke, et al. (2001). "Laryngeal mucosa elasticity and viscosity in high and low relative air humidity." *European Archives of Oto-rhino-laryngology* **258**(3): 125–9.

Herchline, T. and J. K. Amorosa (2002). Tuberculosis, eMedicine. **2002**.

Hidalgo, J. A. and J. A. Vazquez (2002). Candidiasis, eMedicine. **2002**.

Higgins, M. B. and D. H. Chait (1999). "Phonatory air flow characteristics of adductor spasmodic dysphonia and muscle tension dysphonia." *Journal of Speech, Language, and Hearing Research* **42**(1): 101–111.

Hill, J., H. Bird, et al. (2001). "Effect of patient education on adherence to drug treatment for rheumatoid arthritis: A randomised controlled trial." *Ann Rheum Dis* **60**(9): 869–75.

Hilty, D. M., M. Gill, et al. (2002). Hypochondriasis, eMedicine. **2002**.

Hirano, M. (1981). "Structure of the vocal fold in normal and disease states." *Anatomical and Physical Study, America Speech and Hearing Association:* 11–30.

Hirschi, S. D., S. D. Gray, et al. (2002). "Fibronectin: An interesting vocal fold protein." *Journal of Voice* **16**(3): 310–316.

Hodges, N. J. and T. D. Lee (1999). "The role of augmented information prior to learning a bimanual visual-motor coordination task: Do instructions of the movement pattern facilitate learning relative to discovery learning?" *British Journal of Psychology* **90**: 389–403.

Hogikyan, N. D. and G. Sethuraman (1999). "Validation of an instrument to measure voice-related quality of life (V-RQOL)." *J Voice* **13**(4): 557–569.

Hollien, H. (1974). "On vocal registers." *Journal of Phonetics* **2**: 125–143.

Hollien, H., G. T. Girard, et al. (1977). "Vocal fold vibratory patterns of pulse register phonation." *Folia phoniatrica* **29**(3): 200–5.

Holmberg, E. B., R. E. Hillman, et al. (1988). "Glottal airflow and transglottal air pressure measurements for male and female speakers in soft, normal, and loud voice." *The Journal of the Acoustical Society of America* **84**(2): 511–29.

Hsu, K. (2002). Anxiety, eMedicine. **2002**.

Hui, D. S., D. K. Choy, et al. (2001). "Determinants of continuous positive airway pressure compliance in a group of Chinese patients with obstructive sleep apnea." *Chest* **120**(1): 170–6.

Iwarsson, J. (2001). "Effects of inhalatory abdominal wall movement on vertical laryngeal position during phonation." *Journal of Voice* **15**(3): 384–394.

Jacobson, B. H., A. Johnson, et al. (1997). "The voice handicap index (VHI): Development and validation." *American Journal of Speech-Language Pathology* **6**: 66–70.

Jailwala, J. and R. Shaker (2001). Reflux laryngitis, eMedicine. **2002**.

Jiang, J. J. and I. R. Titze (1994). "Measurement of vocal fold intraglottal pressure and impact stress." *Journal of Voice* **8**(2): 132–44.

Jiang, J. J., K. Verdolini, et al. (2000). "Effects of dehydration on phonation in excised canine larynges." *Annals of Otology, Rhinology & Laryngology* **109**(6): 568–575.

Kahn, C. and K. M. Pike (2001). "In search of predictors of dropout from inpatient treatment for anorexia nervosa." *Int J Eat Disord* **30**(3): 237–44.

Kaplan, R. M., C. J. Atkins, et al. (1984). "Specific efficacy expectations mediate exercise compliance in patients with COPD." *Health Psychol* **3**(3): 223–42.

Kaufman, J., R. T. Sataloff, et al. (1996). "Laryngopharyngeal reflux: Consensus conference report." *Journal of Voice* **10**(3): 215–216.

Kaushall, P. I., M. Zetin, et al. (1981). "A psychosocial study of chronic, circumscribed amnesia." *The Journal of Nervous and Mental Disease* **169**(6): 383–389.

Kaye, V. and M. E. Brandsteter (2002). Vertebrobasilar stroke, eMedicine. **2002**.

Kelly, A. H., L. E. Beaton, et al. (1946). "A midbrain mechanism for facio-vocal activity." *Journal of Neurophysiology* **9**: 181–189.

Kelso, J. A. S. (1995). *Dynamic patterns: The self-organization of brain and behavior.* Cambridge, MA: MIT Press.

Kent, R. D., R. L. Sufit, et al. (1991). "Speech deterioration in amyotrophic lateral sclerosis: A case study." *Journal of Speech and Hearing Research* **34**: 1269–1275.

Kent, R. D. (1998). *The speech sciences.* San Diego, CA: Singular Publishing Group, Inc.

Kim, Y. J., A. S. Pakiam, et al. (1999). "Historical and clinical features of psychogenic tremor: A review of 70 cases." *Can J Neurol Sci* **26**(3): 190–195.

Kiortsis, D. N., P. Giral, et al. (2000). "Factors associated with low compliance with lipid-lowering drugs in hyperlipidemic patients." *J Clin Pharm Ther* **25**(6): 445–51.

Kittler, H., R. Weitzdorfer, et al. (2001). "Compliance with follow-up and prognosis among patients with thin melanomas." *Eur J Cancer* **37**(12): 1504–9.

Kjellen, G. and L. Brudin (1994). "Gastroesophageal reflux disease and laryngeal symptoms. Is there really a causal relationship?" *ORL; Journal for Oto-Rhino-Laryngology and Its Related Specialties* **56**: 287–290.

Klapp, S. T. (1977). "Response programming, as assessed by reaction time, does not establish commands for particular muscles." *Journal of Motor Behavior*(9): 301–12.

Koenig, A. S. and S. Jimenez (2002). Scleroderma, eMedicine. **2002**.

Korsch, B. M. and V. F. Negrete (1972). "Doctor-patient communication." *Sci Am* **227**(2): 66–74.

Kotby, M. N., S. R. El-Sady, et al. (1991). "Efficacy of the accent method of voice therapy." *Journal of Voice* **5**(4): 316–320.

Koufman, J. A. (1991). "The otolaryngologic manifestations of gastroesophageal reflux disease (GERD): A clinical investigation of 225 patients using ambulatory 24-hour pH monitoring and an experimental investigation of the role of acid and pepsin in the development of laryngeal injury." *Laryngoscope* **101**(4 Pt 2 Suppl 53): 1–78.

Koufman, J. A. and A. J. Burke (1997). "The etiology and pathogenesis of laryngeal carcinoma." *Otolaryngologic Clinics of North America* **30**(1): 1–19.

Koufman, J. A. and M. M. Cummins (nd.). Prevalence and spectrum of reflux in laryngology: A prospective study of 132 consecutive patents with laryngeal and voice disorders, The Voice Center. **2002**.

Kramer, P. L., D. de Leon, et al. (1990). "Dystonia gene in Askenazi Jewish population is located on chromosome 9q32-34." *Ann Neurol* **2**: 114–120.

Kruse, W., W. Eggert-Kruse, et al. (1993). "Compliance and adverse drug reactions: A prospective study with ethinylestradiol using continuous compliance monitoring." *Clin Investig* **71**(6): 483–7.

Kuna, S. T., J. S. Smickley, et al. (1994). "Cricothyroid muscle activity during sleep in normal adult humans." *Journal of applied physiology* **76**(6): 2326–32.

Landau, M. E. (2001). Conversion disorders, eMedicine. **2002**.

Lane, D., D. Carroll, et al. (2001). "Predictors of attendance at cardiac rehabilitation after myocardial infarction." *J Psychosom Res* **51**(3): 497–501.

Lang, E. and M. Afilalo (2002). Vertebrobasilar atherothrombotic disease, eMedicine. **2002**.

Langkamp, D. L. and S. M. Hlavin (2001). "Factors predicting compliance with palivizumab in high-risk infants." *Am J Perinatol* **18**(6): 345–52.

Larse, L. H. and C. Johnson (2002). Anxiety disorder: Generalized anxiety, eMedicine. **2002**.

Lass, N. J., Ruscello, D. M., Bradshaw, K. H., & Blankenship, B. L. (1991). "Adolescents' perceptions of normal and voice-disordered children." *Journal of Communication Disorders* **24**: 267–274.

Laukkanen, A. (1995). "On speaking voice exercises: A study on the acoustic and physiological effects of speaking voice exercises applying manipulation of the acoustic-aerodynamical state of the supraglottic space and artificially modified auditory feedback (Doctoral dissertation, Tempereen Yliopisto)." *Dissertation Abstracts International* **51**: 207.

Lawrence, V. L. (1978). Medical care for professional voice (panel). *Transcriptions from the Annual Symposium: Care of the Professional Voice*. V. L. Lawrence. New York: The Voice Foundation **3**: 17–18.

Lee, T. D. and E. D. Genovese (1988). "Distribution of practice in motor skill acquisition: Learning and performance effects reconsidered." *Research Quarterly for Exercise and Sport* **59**: 277–287.

Lee, T. D., M. A. White, et al. (1990). "On the role of knowledge of results in motor learning: Exploring the guidance hypothesis." *Journal of Motor Behavior* **22**: 191–208.

Lee, T. D. and S. P. Swinnen (1993). Three legacies of Bryan and Harter: Automaticity, variability and change in skilled performance. *Cognitive issues in motor expertise*. J. L. Starkes and F. Allard. Amsterdam: Elsevier, 295–315.

Lee, T. D., S. P. Swinnen, et al. (1995). "Relative phase alterations during bimanual skill acquisition." *Journal of Motor Behavior* **27**: 263–274.

Lee, T. D. (1998). "On the dynamics of motor learning research." *Res Q Exerc Sport* **69**(4): 334–7.

Lessac, A. (1967). *The use and training of the human voice: A practical approach to speech and voice dynamics.* New York: DBS Publications, Inc.

Lessac, A. (1997). *The use and training of the human voice.* Mt. View, CA: Mayfield Publishing Co.

Liburd, J. D. A. and A. Hebra (2002). Gastroesophageal reflux, eMedicine. **2002**.

Lin, E. H., M. Von Korff, et al. (1995). "The role of the primary care physician in patients' adherence to antidepressant therapy." *Med Care* **33**(1): 67–74.

Linklater, K. (1976). *Freeing the natural voice.* Hollywood, CA: Drama Publishers.

Linville, S. E. (2001). *Vocal aging.* San Diego, CA: Singular.

Lo, R. (1999). "Correlates of expected success at adherence to health regimen of people with IDDM." *J Adv Nurs* **30**(2): 418–24.

Lostao, L., T. E. Joiner, et al. (2001). "Health beliefs and illness attitudes as predictors of breast cancer screening attendance." *Eur J Public Health* **11**(3): 274–9.

Luschei, E. S. (1991). Development of objective standards of nonoral strength and performance: An advocate's view. In: Dysarthria and Apraxia of Speech: Perspectives on Management (C. A. Moore, K. M. Yorkston, & D. R. Beukelman, Eds.). Baltimore: Paul H. Brookes, pp. 173–184.

Marcotullio, D., G. Magliulo, et al. (2002). "Reinke's edema and risk factors: Clinical and histopathologic aspects." *American Journal of Otolaryngology* **23**(2): 81–84.

Marosi, A. and J. Stiesmeyer (2001). "Improving pediatric asthma patient outcomes by incorporation of effective interventions." *J Asthma* **38**(8): 681–90.

Martone, M., N. Butters, et al. (1984). "Dissociations between skill learning and verbal recognition in amnesia and dementia." *Archives of Neurology* **41**: 965–970.

Matsumoto, J. Y. (1996). Surface electromyographic studies of movement disorders. In: Clinical Neurophysiology (Daube, J. R., ed). F.A. Davis Company: Philadelphia, PA, pp 341–353.

Maviglia, S. M., J. M. Teich, et al. (2001). "Using an electronic medical record to identify opportunities to improve compliance with cholesterol guidelines." *J Gen Intern Med* **16**(8): 531–7.

McArdle, W. D., F. I. Katch, et al. (1996). *Exercise physiology: Energy, nutrition, and human performance.* Baltimore, MD: Williams & Wilkins.

McAuley, J., and Rothwell, J. (2004). "Identification of psychogenic, dystonic, and other organic tremors by a coherence entrainment test." *Movement Disorders* **19**(3):253–267.

McAuley, E., H. M. Talbot, et al. (1999). "Manipulating self-efficacy in the exercise environment in women: Influences on affective responses." *Health Psychol* **18**(3): 288–94.

McClay, J. E. (2001). Subglottic stenosis in children, eMedicine. **2002**.

McNeil, B. K., H. Guinto-Ocampo, et al. (2002). Pertussis, eMedicine. **2002**.

McNevin, N. H., C. H. Shea, et al. (2001). "Increasing the distance of an external focus of attention enhances learning." *Psychological Research* **67**(1): 22–29.

Mehta, R. P., S. N. Goldman, & Orloff, L. A. (2001). "Long-term therapy for spasmodic dysphonia: Acoustic and aerodynamic outcomes." *Arch Otolaryngol Head Neck Surg* **127**(4): 393–399.

Mercante, G., A. Bacciu, et al. (2003). "Gastroesophageal reflux as a possible co-promoting factor in the development of the squamous-cell carcinoma of the oral cavity, of the larynx and of the pharynx." *Acta Oto-Rhino-Laryngologica Belgica* **57**(2): 113–117.

Milanov, I. (2001). "Electromyographic differentiation of tremors." *Clinical Neurophysiology* **112**: 1626–1632.

Milanov, I. (2002). "Clinical and electromyographic examinations of patients with psychogenic tremor." *Electromyogr Clin Neurophysiol* **42**(7): 387–392.

Miller, L. J. (1990). "The formal treatment contract in the inpatient management of borderline personality disorder." *Hosp Community Psychiatry* **41**(9): 985–7.

Moon, J. B. and D. L. Jones (1991). "Motor control of velopharyngeal structures during vowel production." *Cleft Palate Craniofac J* **28**(3): 267–73.

Morgan, K., J. Thompson, et al. (2003). "Predicting longer-term outcomes following psychological treatment for hypnotic-dependent chronic insomnia." *J Psychosom Res* **54**(1): 21–9.

Morrison, M., L. Rammage, et al. (1999). "The irritable larynx syndrome." *Journal of Voice* **13**(3): 447–455.

Munhall, K. G., A. Lofqvist, et al. (1994). "Lip-larynx coordination in speech: Effects of mechanical perturbations to the lower lip." *J Acoust Soc Am* **95**(6): 3605–16.

Muñiz, A. (2002). Croup, eMedicine. **2002**.

Neely, J. H. (1977). "Semantic priming and retrieval from lexical memory: Roles of inhibitionless spreading activation and limited-capacity attention." *Journal of Experimental Psychology: General* **106**(3): 226–254.

Neily, J. B., K. H. Toto, et al. (2002). "Potential contributing factors to noncompliance with dietary sodium restriction in patients with heart failure." *Am Heart J* **143**(1): 29–33.

Olson, K. (1999). Spasmodic dysphonia, Grand Rounds Archive at Baylor. **2003**.

Pan, W. H., H. Y. Chang, et al. (2001). "Prevalence, awareness, treatment and control of hypertension in Taiwan: Results of nutrition and health survey in Taiwan (NAHSIT) 1993–1996." *J Hum Hypertens* **15**(11): 793–8.

Pang, S. K., W. Y. Ip, et al. (2001). "Psychosocial correlates of fluid compliance among Chinese haemodialysis patients." *J Adv Nurs* **35**(5): 691–8.

Parker, J. J., K. P. Fennelly, et al. (1998). "Irritant-associated vocal cord dysfunction." *Journal of Occupational and Environmental Medicine* **40**(2): 136–143.

Patti, M., U. Diener, et al. (2002). Gastroesophageal reflux diseases, eMedicine. **2002**.

Paulson, G. W. (1997). Meige's syndrome. **2003**.

Pawlak, A. S., T. Hammond, et al. (1996). "Immunocytochemical study of proteoglycans in vocal folds." *Annals of Otology, Rhinology, and Laryngology* **105**(1): 6–11.

Pert, C. B. (1997). *Molecules of emotion: The science behind mind-body medicine.* New York: Touchstone.

Peterson, K. L., K. Verdolini-Marston, et al. (1994). "Comparison of aerodynamic and electroglottographic parameters in evaluating clinically relevant voicing patterns." *Annals of Otology, Rhinology, and Laryngology* **103**(5 Pt. 1): 335–346.

Polenakovik, H. (2002). Actinomycosis, eMedicine. **2002**.

Porras Alonso, E., A. Martin Mateos, et al. (2002). "Laryngeal tuberculosis." *Rev Laryngol Otol Rhinol (Bord)* **123**(1): 47–8.

Protagoras-Lianos, D. (2001). Somatoform disorder: Pain, eMedicine. **2002**.

Raethjena, R., Pawlasa, F., Lindemanna, M., Wenzelburgera, R., & Deuschl, G. (2000). "Determinants of physiologic tremor in a large normal population." *Clinical Neurophysiology* **111**:1825–1837.

Ramig, L. O., R. C. Scherer, et al. (1990). "Acoustic analysis of voice in amyotrophic lateral sclerosis: A longitudinal case study." *Journal of Speech and Hearing Disorders* **55**: 2–14.

Ramig, L. O., S. Countryman, et al. (1996). "Intensive speech treatment for patients with Parkinson's disease: Short-and long-term comparison of two techniques." *Neurology* **47**(6): 1496–1504.

Rawl, S. M., V. L. Champion, et al. (2000). "The impact of age and race on mammography practices." *Health Care Women Int* **21**(7): 583–97.

Reynolds, S. A., M. W. Schmid, et al. (2004). "Polydipsia screening tool." *Archives of Psychiatric Nursing* **XVIII**(2): 49–59.

Reynolds, S. A., M. W. Schmid, et al. (2004). "Identifying at risk nursing home residents using a polydipsia screening tool." *Archives of Psychiatric Nursing* **XVIII**(2): 60–67.

Richter, B., E. Lohle, et al. (2000). "Working conditions on the stage: Climatic considerations." *Logoped Phoniatr Vocol* **25**: 80–86.

Richter, B., E. Lohle, et al. (2002). "Harmful substances on the opera stage: Possible negative effects on singers' respiratory tracts." *Journal of Voice* **16**(1): 72–80.

Robin, D. A., Goel, A., Somodi, L. B., & Luschei, E. S. (1992). "Tongue strength and endurance: Relation to highly skilled movements." *Journal of Speech and Hearing Research* **35**: 1239–1245.

Roediger, H. L. (1990). "Implicit memory." *American Psychologist* **45**(9): 1043–1056.

Rosen, D. C. and R. T. Sataloff (1997). *Psychology of voice disorders*. San Diego, CA: Singular Publishing Group, Inc.

Rosen, C. A. (2002). Vocal fold paralysis, unilateral, eMedicine. **2002**.

Ross, M. A., R. G. Miller, et al. (1998). "Toward earlier diagnosis of amyotrophic lateral sclerosis." *Neurology* **50**(3): 768–772.

Roto, P. and E. Sala (1996). "Occupational laryngitis caused by formaldehyde: A case report." *American Journal of Industrial Medicine* **29**: 275–277.

Roy, N. and H. A. Leeper (1993). "Effects of the manual laryngeal musculo-skeletal tension reduction technique as a treatment for functional voice disorders: Perceptual and acoustic measures." *Journal of Voice* **7**: 242–249.

Roy, N., C. N. Ford, et al. (1996). "Muscle tension dysphonia and spasmodic dysphonia: The role of manual laryngeal tension reduction in diagnosis and management." *Annals of Otology, Rhinology, and Laryngology* **105**(11): 851–856.

Roy, N., D. M. Bless, et al. (1997). "Manual circumlaryngeal therapy for functional dysphonia: An evaluation of short- and long-term treatment outcomes." *Journal of Voice* **11**: 321–331.

Roy, N., D. M. Bless, et al. (2000a). "Personality and voice disorders: A multitrait-multidisorder analysis." *J Voice* **14**(4): 521–548.

Roy, N., D. M. Bless, et al. (2000b). "Personality and voice disorders: A super-factor trait analysis." *J Speech Lang Hear Res* **43**(3): 749–768.

Roy, N., S. D. Gray, et al. (2001). "An evaluation of the effects of two treatment approaches for teachers with voice disorders: A prospective randomized clinical trial." *Journal of Speech, Language, and Hearing Research* **44**(2): 286–296.

Ruscello, D. M., Lass, N. J., & Podbesek, J. (1988). "Listeners' perceptions of normal and voice-disordered children." *Folia Phoniatrica* **40**:290–296.

Russo-Magno, P., A. O'Brien, et al. (2001). "Compliance with CPAP therapy in older men with obstructive sleep apnea." *J Am Geriatr Soc* **49**(9): 1205–11.

Sabol, J. W., L. Lee, et al. (1995). "The value of vocal function exercises in the practice regimen of singers." *Journal of Voice* **9**(1): 27–36.

Safren, S. A., M. W. Otto, et al. (2001). "Two strategies to increase adherence to HIV antiretroviral medication: Life-steps and medication monitoring." *Behav Res Ther* **39**(10): 1151–62.

Sala, E., M. Hytonen, et al. (1996). "Occupational laryngitis with immediate allergic or immediate type specified chemical hypersensitivity." *Clin Otolaryngol* **21**(1): 42–48.

Salmon, B. (2001). "Differences between men and women in compliance with risk factor reduction: Before and after coronary artery bypass surgery." *J Vasc Nurs* **19**(3): 73–77.

Salomone, J. A. I. (2004). Dehydration in adults. *Environmental exposures and injuries.* S. H. Plantz, F. Talavera and S. L. Bernstein. **2004**.

Sanders, I. and L. Mu (1998). "Anatomy of the human internal superior laryngeal nerve." *The Anatomical Record* **252**(4): 646–56.

Sapienza, C. M., M. A. Crary, et al. (1996). "Laryngeal aerodynamic aspects of women with adductor spasmodic dysphonia." *Arch Otolaryngol Head Neck Surg* **122**(4): 385–388.

Sapienza, C. M., M. P. Cannito, et al. (2002). "Acoustic variations in reading produced by speakers with spasmodic dysphonia pre-botox injection and within early stages of post-botox injection." *J Speech Lang Hear Res* **45**(5): 830–843.

Sappok, T., A. Faulstich, et al. (2001). "Compliance with secondary prevention of ischemic stroke: A prospective evaluation." *Stroke* **32**(8): 1884–9.

Sataloff, R. T. (1987). "The professional voice: Part III. Common diagnoses and treatments." *Journal of Voice* **1**(3): 283–292.

Sataloff, R. T. (1987). "The professional voice: Part I. Anatomy, function, and general health." *Journal of Voice* **1**(1): 92–104.

Sataloff, R. T., B. C. Baron, et al. (1988). "Discussion: Acute medical problems of the voice." *Journal of Voice* **2**(4): 345–353.

Sataloff, R. T. (1992). "The impact of pollution on the voice." *Otolaryngology Head and Neck Surgery* **106**: 701–705.

Sataloff, R. T. (1997). *Professional voice: The science and art of clinical.* San Diego, Singular Publishing Group, Inc.

Scherer, Y. K. and S. Bruce (2001). "Knowledge, attitudes, and self-efficacy and compliance with medical regimen, number of emergency department visits, and hospitalizations in adults with asthma." *Heart Lung* **30**(4): 250–7.

Schmidt, R. A. and G. Wulf (1997). "Continuous concurrent feedback degrades skill learning: Implications for training and simulation." *Hum Factors* **39**(4): 509–25.

Schmidt, R. A. and T. D. Lee (1999). *Motor control and learning.* Champaign, IL: Human Kinetics.

Services, U. S. D. o. H. a. H. (1985). *The health consequences of smoking: Cancer and chronic diseases in the workplace; a report of the Surgeon General.* Washington, DC: U.S. Government Printing Office.

Shah, A. K. (2002). Myasthenia Gravis, eMedicine. **2002**.

Sharma, S. (2002). Pneumonia, bacterial, eMedicine. **2002**.

Sharma, S. and G. Thomson (2002). Wegener granulomatosis, eMedicine. **2002**.

Shaw, G. Y., J. P. Searl, et al. (1996). "Subjective, laryngoscopic, and acoustic measures of laryngeal reflux before and after treatment with omeprazol." *Journal of Voice* **10**(4): 410–418.

Shaw, G. Y. and J. P. Searl (1997). "Laryngeal manifestations of gastroesophageal reflux before and after treatment with omeprazole." *Southern Medical Journal* **90**: 1115–1122.

Shea, C. H. and G. Wulf (1999). "Enhancing motor learning through external-focus instructions and feedback." *Human Movement Science* **18**: 553–571.

Shemesh, E., A. Rudnick, et al. (2001). "A prospective study of posttraumatic stress symptoms and nonadherence in survivors of a myocardial infarction (MI)." *Gen Hosp Psychiatry* **23**(4): 215–22.

Silverman, R. S., T. L. Lee-Chiong, Jr., et al. (1995). "Stridor from edema of the arytenoids, epiglottis, and vocal cords after use of free-base cocaine." *Chest* **108**(5): 1477–8.

Sivasankar, M. and K. V. Fisher (2002). "Oral breathing increases Ph and vocal effort by superficial drying of vocal fold mucosa." *Journal of Voice* **16**(2): 172–181.

Sivasankar, M. and K. V. Fisher (2003). "Oral breathing challenge in participants with vocal attrition." *Journal of Speech-Language-Hearing Research* **46**(6): 1416–1427.

Smaga, S. (2003). "Tremor." *Am Fam Physician* **68**: 1545–53.

Smith, S. and K. Thyme (1978). *Accent Metoden*. Herning, Denmark: Special Paedagogisk Forlag.

Sobol, S. E., M. D. Schloss, et al. (2002). Sinusitis, acute, medical treatment, eMedicine. **2002**.

Soreff, S. and L. A. McInnes (2002). Bipolar affective disorder, eMedicine. **2002**.

Speaks, C. E. (1999). *Introduction to sound: Acoustics for the hearing and speech sciences*. San Diego, CA: Singular Publishing Group, Inc.

Spears, N. M., R. A. Leadbetter, et al. (1996). "Clozapine treatment in polydipsia and intermittent hyponatremia." *Journal of Clinical Psychiatry* **57**(3): 123–128.

Spiegel, J. R., M. Hawkshaw, et al. (2000). "Dysphonia related to medical therapy." *Otolaryngol Clin North Am* **33**(4): 771–84.

Stager, S., Bielamowicz, S., Regnell, J. R., Gupta, A., & Barkmeier, J. (2000). "Supraglottic activity: Evidence of vocal hyperfunction or laryngeal articulation?" *Journal of Speech, Language, and Hearing Research* **43**(1): 229–238.

Steinhauer, K. and J. P. Grayhack (2000). "The role of knowledge of results in performance and learning of a voice motor task." *J Voice* **14**(2): 137–45.

Stemple, J. C., L. Lee, et al. (1994). "Efficacy of vocal function exercises as a method of improving voice production." *Journal of Voice* **8**(3): 271–278.

Story, B. H., I. R. Titze, et al. (1998). "Vocal tract functions for an adult female speaker based on volumetric imaging." *The Journal of the Acoustical Society of America* **104**(1): 471–487.

Strand, E. A., E. H. Buder, et al. (1993). "Differential phonatory characteristics of women with amyotrophic lateral sclerosis." *NCVS Status and Progress Report* **4**: 151–167.

Strum, S. (2001). Overuse injury, eMedicine. **2002**.

Sundberg, J. (1977). "The acoustics of the singing voice." *Scientific American:* 82–91.

Swinnen, S. P. and R. G. Carson (2002). "The control and learning of patterns of interlimb coordination: Past and present issues in normal and disordered control." *Acta Psychol (Amst)* **110**(2–3): 129–37.

Takanokura, M., Kokuzawa, N., & Sakamoto, K. (2002). "The origins of physiological tremor as deduced from immersions of the finger in various liquids." *Eur J Appl Physiol* **88**: 29–41.

Takanokura, M. and Sakamoto, K. (2001). "Physiological tremor of the upper limb segments." *Eur J Appl Physiol* **85**: 214–25.

Taylor, D. W., D. L. Sackett, et al. (1978). "Compliance with antihypertensive drug therapy." *Ann N Y Acad Sci* **304**: 390–403.

Taylor, R. F. and G. R. Bernard (1989). "Airway complications from free-basing cocaine." *Chest* **95**(2): 476–7.

Thawley, S. E., W. R. Panje, et al. (1987). *Comprehensive management of head and neck tumors*. Philadelphia, PA: W.B. Saunders Company.

Titze, I. R. (1981). Heat generation in the vocal folds and its possible effect on vocal endurance. *Transcripts of the tenth symposium: Care of the professional voice. Part 1: Instrumentation in voice research.* V. L. Lawrence. New York: The Voice Foundation, 52–65.

Titze, I. R. (1988). "The physics of small-amplitude oscillation of the vocal folds." *The Journal of the Acoustical Society of America* **83**(4): 1536–52.

Titze, I. R. (1994). *Principles of voice production*. Englewood Cliffs, NJ: Prentice-Hall.

Titze, I. R. and B. H. Story (1997). "Acoustic interactions of the voice source with the lower vocal tract." *J Acoust Soc Am* **101**(4): 2234–43.

Tranel, D., A. R. Damasio, et al. (1994). "Sensorimotor skill learning in amnesia: Additional evidence for the neural basis of nondeclarative memory." *Learning and Memory* **1**(3): 165–179.

Tucker, C. M., R. S. Fennell, et al. (2002). "Associations with medication adherence among ethnically different pediatric patients with renal transplants." *Pediatr Nephrol* **17**(4): 251–6.

Turvey, M. T. (1990). "Coordination." *Am Psychol* **45**(8): 938–53.

Vakil, E., L. Grunhaus, et al. (2000). "The effect of electroconvulsive therapy (ECT) on implicit memory: Skill learning and perceptual priming in patients with major depression." *Neuropsychologia* **38**(10): 1405–1414.

Valtin, H. (2002). "'Drink at least eight glasses of water a day.' Really? Is there scientific evidence for '8 X 8'?" *American Journal of Physiology. Regulatory, Integrative and Comparative Physiology* **283**: R993–R1004.

van der Palen, J., J. J. Klein, et al. (2001). "Behavioural effect of self-treatment guidelines in a self-management program for adults with asthma." *Patient Educ Couns* **43**(2): 161–9.

van Es, S. M., A. F. Nagelkerke, et al. (2001). "An intervention programme using the ASE-model aimed at enhancing adherence in adolescents with asthma." *Patient Educ Couns* **44**(3): 193–203.

Vander Linden, D. W., J. H. Cauraugh, et al. (1993). "The effect of frequency of kinetic feedback on learning an isometric force production task in nondisabled subjects." *Physical Therapy* **73**: 79–87.

Varkey, B. and A. B. Varkey (2002). Pneumonia, aspiration, eMedicine. **2002**.

Verdolini, K. (1988). "Practice good vocal health and prevent those voice disorders." *Choristers Guild Lett*(2): 40–44.

Verdolini, K., I. R. Titze, et al. (1994). "Dependence of phonatory effort on hydration level." *Journal of Speech and Hearing Research* **37**(5): 1001–7.

Verdolini, K., M. Sandage, et al. (1994). "Effaced of hydration treatments on laryngeal nodules and polyps and related voice measures." *Journal of Voice* **8**(1): 30–47.

Verdolini, K., D. G. Druker, et al. (1998). "Laryngeal adduction in resonant voice." *Journal of Voice* **12**(3): 315–327.

Verdolini, K. and D. Krebs (1999). Some considerations on the science of special challenges in voice training. *Voice tradition and technology: A state-of-the-art studio*. G. Nair. San Diego, CA: Singular Publishing Group, Inc., 227–239.

Verdolini, K. and L. O. Ramig (2001). "Review: Occupational risks for voice problems." *Logoped Phoniatr Vocol* **26**(1): 37–46.

Verdolini, K., Y. Min, et al. (2002). "Biological mechanisms underlying voice changes due to dehydration." *Journal of Speech, Language, and Hearing Research* **45**: 268–281.

Verdolini-Marston, K., Y. Min, et al. (1990). "Changes in phonation threshold pressure with induced conditions of hydration." *Journal of Voice* **4**(2): 142–151.

Verdolini-Marston, K., M. Sandage, et al. (1994). "Effect of hydration treatments on laryngeal nodules and polyps and related voice measures." *Journal of Voice* **8**(1): 30–47.

Ward, P. D., S. L. Thibeault, et al. (2002). "Hyaluronic acid: Its role in voice." *Journal of Voice* **16**(3): 303–309.

Werning, J., L. McAllister, et al. (nd.). Functional voice disorders, emedicine. **2003**.

Wheatley, J. R., A. Brancatisano, et al. (1991). "Respiratory-related activity of cricothyroid muscle in awake normal humans." *Journal of Applied Physiology* **70**(5): 2226–32.

Wilbourn, A. J. (1994). "Clinical neurophysiology in the diagnosis of amyotrophic lateral sclerosis: The Lambert and the El Escorial criteria." *Journal of Neurological Sciences* **124 Suppl**: 96–107.

Winfield, J. (2002). Fibromyalgia, eMedicine. **2002**.

Winstein, C. J. and R. A. Schmidt (1990). "Reduced frequency of knowledge of results enhances motor skill learning." *Journal of Experimental Psychology: Learning, Memory, and Cognition* **16**: 677–691.

Woodson, G. E. (1993). "Configuration of the glottis in laryngeal paralysis II: Animal experiments." *Laryngoscope* **103**(11 Part 1): 1235–1241.

Woodson, G. E., M. P. Murry, et al. (1998). "Unilateral cricothyroid contraction and glottic configuration." *Journal of Voice* **12**(3): 335–9.

Yates, W. R. (2002). Somatoform disorders, eMedicine. **2002**.

Zemlin, W. R. (1998). *Speech and hearing science anatomy and physiology.* Boston: Allyn and Bacon.

Zola-Morgan, S., L. R. Squire, et al. (1982). "The neuroanatomy of amnesia: Amygdala-hippocampus versus temporal stem." *Science* **218**(4579): 1337–1339.

Author Index

279